Pediatric Bleeding Disorders

Amy L. Dunn • Bryce A. Kerlin
Sarah H. O'Brien • Melissa J. Rose
Riten Kumar
Editors

Pediatric Bleeding Disorders

A Clinical Casebook

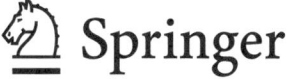

Editors
Amy L. Dunn, MD
Division of Pediatric Hematology
Oncology and Bone Marrow
Transplant
Nationwide Children's Hospital
Columbus, OH
USA

Bryce A. Kerlin, MD
Division of Pediatric Hematology
Oncology and Bone Marrow
Transplant
Nationwide Children's Hospital
Columbus, OH
USA

Sarah H. O'Brien, MD
Division of Pediatric Hematology
Oncology and Bone Marrow
Transplant
Nationwide Children's Hospital
Columbus, OH
USA

Melissa J. Rose, DO
Division of Pediatric Hematology
Oncology and Bone Marrow
Transplant
Nationwide Children's Hospital
Columbus, OH
USA

Riten Kumar, MD, MSc
Division of Pediatric Hematology
Oncology and Bone Marrow
Transplant
Nationwide Children's Hospital
Columbus, OH
USA

ISBN 978-3-030-31660-0   ISBN 978-3-030-31661-7 (eBook)
https://doi.org/10.1007/978-3-030-31661-7

© Springer Nature Switzerland AG 2020

This work is subject to copyright. All rights are reserved by the Publisher, whether the whole or part of the material is concerned, specifically the rights of translation, reprinting, reuse of illustrations, recitation, broadcasting, reproduction on microfilms or in any other physical way, and transmission or information storage and retrieval, electronic adaptation, computer software, or by similar or dissimilar methodology now known or hereafter developed.

The use of general descriptive names, registered names, trademarks, service marks, etc. in this publication does not imply, even in the absence of a specific statement, that such names are exempt from the relevant protective laws and regulations and therefore free for general use.

The publisher, the authors and the editors are safe to assume that the advice and information in this book are believed to be true and accurate at the date of publication. Neither the publisher nor the authors or the editors give a warranty, expressed or implied, with respect to the material contained herein or for any errors or omissions that may have been made. The publisher remains neutral with regard to jurisdictional claims in published maps and institutional affiliations.

This Springer imprint is published by the registered company Springer Nature Switzerland AG
The registered company address is: Gewerbestrasse 11, 6330 Cham, Switzerland

Preface

When this book was conceived, the editors were partners at Nationwide Children's Hospital in Columbus, Ohio. The editors share a lifelong passion for clinical pediatric hemostasis, along with a similar passion for mentorship and education. We also realize the value of having partners and friends who share our interests. The field of pediatric hemostasis has evolved dramatically over the last decade as new interventions such as gene therapy, antibody-based therapies, and cellular therapies become realities; significant time and effort must be dedicated to learning about how and when to use these options. In addition, hemostasis testing is evolving, and increasingly, knowledge about the power of genetic testing and global hemostatic assays is vitally important. Categorical clinical training schedules, however, have increasing demands because every aspect of hematology, oncology, and bone marrow transplant is complex and rapidly evolving. For this reason, Dr. Bryce A. Kerlin had the vision to create a fourth year hemostasis/thrombosis fellowship to meet the training needs of future generations of pediatric hemostasis physicians. The fellowship provides 1–2 years of protected time, individualized to the trainee's wants and needs. It also provides the opportunity to travel to relevant meetings such as the American Society of Hematology, Hemophilia Academy, and the Hemostasis and Thrombosis Research Society annual meetings. Our fellows have benefitted from these meetings to develop their own relationships and collaborators in the field. Fortunately, a local benefactor, Ms. Joan Wallick shared Dr. Kerlin's vision, and our fellowship is endowed in her name. Our team has benefitted enormously from the excitement and enthusiasm of our trainees, and we have all grown because of this program. The fellows have all produced important and impactful academic works on a variety of hemostasis related projects.

As the editors planned this book, we decided to merge our passions for hemostasis and mentorship. Each editor paired with a former fellow who had completed either a categorical or fourth year fellowship with us. Each pair aimed to create clinical vignettes that would be approachable and illustrative of common scenarios encountered in pediatric hematology practice. The aim was to work through a differential diagnosis and initial treatment approach to each scenario and to offer a few clinical pearls at the end of each chapter. As so often happens in academic life, this group of collaborators no longer all work in the same city, but the collaborations, mentoring, and friendships continue despite physical distance. We dedicate this book to the generosity of Ms. Wallick, the spirit of mentorship, the patients and families who inspire us to keep learning, and all those who love the clinical conundrums associated with a vibrant pediatric hemostasis-thrombosis program.

Columbus, OH, USA

Amy L. Dunn, MD
Bryce A. Kerlin, MD
Sarah H. O'Brien, MD
Melissa J. Rose, DO
Riten Kumar, MD, MSc

Contents

Part I Hemophilia A and B

1 **Management of an Infant with Hemophilia A** 3
   Surbhi Saini and Amy L. Dunn

2 **Clinical Care of a Child with Hemophilia A
   and Inhibitors** 13
   Surbhi Saini and Amy L. Dunn

3 **Diagnosis and Management of a Patient with
   Newly Diagnosed Hemophilia B** 25
   Surbhi Saini and Amy L. Dunn

4 **Approach to a Child with Hemophilia B
   and Anaphylaxis to Factor IX** 35
   Surbhi Saini and Amy L. Dunn

Part II Rare Factor Deficiencies

5 **Manifestations and Treatment of Congenital
   Fibrinogen Deficiency**.......................... 51
   Ruchika Sharma and Bryce A. Kerlin

6 **Diagnosis and Management of FVII Deficiency**..... 59
   Ruchika Sharma and Bryce A. Kerlin

7 **Approach to Mucosal Bleeding in an Adolescent
   with FXI Deficiency** 65
   Ruchika Sharma and Bryce A. Kerlin

8	**Recognition and Care of a Newborn with FXIII Deficiency** 71
	Bryce A. Kerlin

Part III von Willebrand Disease

9	**Classification and Management of Type 1 von Willebrand Disease** 83
	Dominder Kaur and Sarah H. O'Brien

10	**Presentation and Management of Type 2 von Willebrand Disease** 99
	Dominder Kaur and Sarah H. O'Brien

11	**Clinical Approach to Type 3 von Willebrand Disease** 113
	Dominder Kaur and Sarah H. O'Brien

12	**Pathophysiology and Management of Acquired von Willebrand Syndrome** 127
	Dominder Kaur and Sarah H. O'Brien

Part IV Thrombocytopenias

13	**Approach to a Patient with Sudden Onset of Mucocutaneous Bleeding and Thrombocytopenia** ... 141
	Melissa J. Rose and Amanda Jacobson-Kelly

14	**A Preteen Female with Fatigue and Incidental Finding of Thrombocytopenia** 151
	Melissa J. Rose and Amanda Jacobson-Kelly

15	**Diagnosis and Management of an Infant with Microthrombocytopenia** 161
	Melissa J. Rose and Amanda Jacobson-Kelly

16	**Care of a Toddler with Epistaxis and Bernard-Soulier Syndrome** 171
	Melissa J. Rose and Amanda Jacobson-Kelly

Part V Platelet Dysfunctions

17 Caring for an Infant with Heelstick Bleeding 185
Gary M. Woods and Riten Kumar

18 Approach to a Child with Epistaxis and Macrothrombocytopenia 195
Gary M. Woods and Riten Kumar

19 Recognition and Management of Congenital Platelet Granule Disorders 205
Gary M. Woods and Riten Kumar

Index 219

Contributors

Amy L. Dunn, MD Nationwide Children's Hospital, Division of Pediatric Hematology, Oncology and Bone Marrow Transplant, Columbus, OH, USA

Department of Pediatrics, The Ohio State University College of Medicine, Columbus, OH, USA

Amanda Jacobson-Kelly, MD Nationwide Children's Hospital, Division of Pediatric Hematology, Oncology and Bone Marrow Transplant, Columbus, OH, USA

Department of Pediatrics, The Ohio State University College of Medicine, Columbus, OH, USA

Dominder Kaur, MD Department of Pediatrics, Division of Pediatric Hematology/Oncology/Stem Cell Transplant, Columbia University Irving Medical Center, Children's Hospital of New York/New York Presbyterian Morgan Stanley Children's Hospital, New York, NY, USA

Bryce A. Kerlin, MD Nationwide Children's Hospital, Division of Pediatric Hematology, Oncology and Bone Marrow Transplant, Columbus, OH, USA

Department of Pediatrics, The Ohio State University College of Medicine, Columbus, OH, USA

Center for Clinical and Translational Research, Abigail Wexner Research Institute, Columbus, OH, USA

Riten Kumar, MD, MSc Nationwide Children's Hospital, Division of Pediatric Hematology, Oncology and Bone Marrow Transplant, Columbus, OH, USA

Department of Pediatrics, The Ohio State University College of Medicine, Columbus, OH, USA

Sarah H. O'Brien, MD Nationwide Children's Hospital, Division of Pediatric Hematology, Oncology and Bone Marrow Transplant, Columbus, OH, USA

Center for Innovation in Pediatric Practice, Abigail Wexner Research Institute at Nationwide Children's Hospital, Columbus, OH, USA

Department of Pediatrics, The Ohio State University College of Medicine, Columbus, OH, USA

Melissa J. Rose, DO Nationwide Children's Hospital, Division of Pediatric Hematology, Oncology and Bone Marrow Transplant, Columbus, OH, USA

Department of Pediatrics, The Ohio State University College of Medicine, Columbus, OH, USA

Surbhi Saini, MD Department of Pediatrics, St. Louis Children's Hospital, St. Louis, MO, USA

Washington University in St. Louis School of Medicine, St. Louis, MO, USA

Ruchika Sharma, MD Medical College of Wisconsin, Versiti Wisconsin, Milwaukee, WI, USA

Gary M. Woods, MD Division of Hematology/Oncology/BMT, Children's Healthcare of Atlanta, Atlanta, GA, USA

Department of Pediatrics, Emory University School of Medicine, Atlanta, GA, USA

Part I

Hemophilia A and B

Management of an Infant with Hemophilia A

Surbhi Saini and Amy L. Dunn

Case Presentation You are called to the newborn nursery to consult on a 2-day-old male with circumcision-related bleeding. You find a term infant who was born by spontaneous vaginal delivery. There is no family history of bleeding disorders, and the mother was taking no medications during the pregnancy. He received vitamin K at birth. On physical examination, he is a well-developed, non-dysmorphic infant. His anterior fontanelle is flat. He has mild pallor and oozing from his circumcision site. He has no bruising or petechia. His vital signs are normal for age.

S. Saini
Department of Pediatrics, St. Louis Children's Hospital, St. Louis, MO, USA

Washington University in St. Louis School of Medicine, St. Louis, MO, USA

A. L. Dunn (✉)
Nationwide Children's Hospital, Division of Pediatric Hematology, Oncology and Bone Marrow Transplant, Columbus, OH, USA

Department of Pediatrics, The Ohio State University College of Medicine, Columbus, OH, USA
e-mail: amy.dunn@nationwidechildrens.org

© Springer Nature Switzerland AG 2020
A. L. Dunn et al. (eds.), *Pediatric Bleeding Disorders*,
https://doi.org/10.1007/978-3-030-31661-7_1

Multiple-Choice Management Question

You suspect that this child has a congenital bleeding disorder. Do you:

A. Give fresh frozen plasma
B. Give cryoprecipitate
C. Call for a STAT hematology consult

Differential Diagnosis

The differential in this infant includes congenital factor deficiencies, severe Von Willebrand disease, hypo-/dysfibrinogenemia, thrombocytopenia, disseminated intravascular coagulation, liver disease, vitamin K deficiency, and platelet dysfunction (Fig. 1.1).

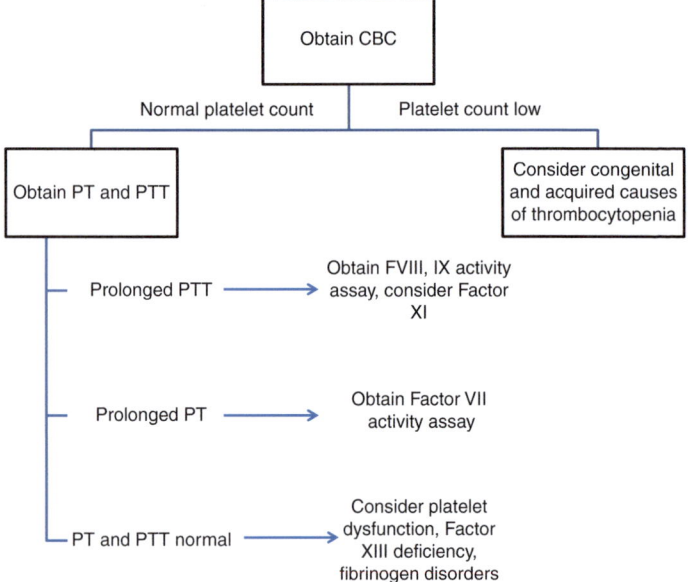

Fig. 1.1 A laboratory approach to the differential diagnosis in a healthy, male infant with prolonged bleeding from circumcision. *CBC* complete blood count, *PT* protime, *PTT* activated partial thromboplastin time

Management

Our patient has persistent, mild oozing but is clinically stable. This allows time to evaluate him and work through the differential diagnosis.

Laboratory Findings

A normal protime (PT), platelet count, fibrinogen, and thrombin time along with an elevated partial thromboplastin time (aPTT) and decreased plasma FVIII activity assay confirm the diagnosis of hemophilia A. Communication with the special coagulation laboratory is crucial to ensure timely and accurate laboratory results. The reagents necessary to perform factor VIII and FIX assays are expensive, and these assays require technical expertise. A call to the laboratory informing them of a suspected diagnosis of hemophilia will enable the laboratory to return results in the most expeditious fashion. Type 3 VWD, which can present in a similar way with elevated aPTT and decreased plasma FVIII levels, needs to be differentiated from hemophilia A. Patients with type 3 VWD will have absent multimers, along with low FVIII, VWF antigen, and ristocetin cofactor activity. VWD Normandy variant (type 2 N), which results from decreased FVIII binding to Von Willebrand factor should also be considered in the setting of moderately low FVIII levels or an autosomal inheritance pattern. This can be evaluated with a FVIII binding assay and VWD mutation analysis.

Diagnosis and Assessment

Hemophilia A, or "classic hemophilia," is a congenital bleeding disorder that results from congenital deficiency or absence of circulating factor VIII (FVIII). It is an X-linked recessive disorder with an incidence of approximately 1:5000 male births [1]. Hemophilia B is also X-linked and has an incidence of 1:20,000 male births. Hemophilia is found across the globe and affects every racial and ethnic group.

Factor VIII is a 320 kilodalton glycoprotein that is produced predominantly in the liver sinusoidal endothelial cells. Factor VIII

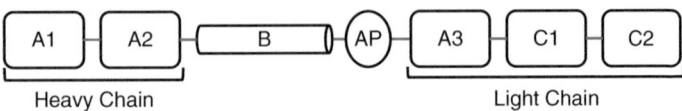

Fig. 1.2 Factor VIII consists of three A domains, one B domain, and two C domains that are linked by an activation peptide (AP)

consists of six domains, A1-A2-B-A3-C1-C2 (Fig. 1.2) with the encoding gene found on the long arm of the X chromosome (Xq28). Upon release into the circulation, FVIII is non-covalently linked to Von Willebrand factor (VWF). VWF protects FVIII from degradation and increases the circulatory half-life from approximately 2 to 12 hours. Upon activation, FVIII is released from VWF, and the activated factor VIIIa acts as a cofactor in the activation of factor X by factor IXa on the surface of activated platelets.

The most common bleeding manifestations in hemophilia A are delayed bleeding, and joint and muscle bleeding. In the newborn period, the most common symptoms are bleeding from circumcision, heel sticks, oral mucosa, and, rarely, intracranial hemorrhage [2]. Therefore, infants born to known carrier mothers should not be circumcised until FVIII or IX activity assay results rule out hemophilia. Nonetheless, lack of bleeding with circumcision does not rule out hemophilia as the incidence of circumcision-related bleeding is reported to be 23–48.2% [3, 4]. Additionally, a lack of family history does not eliminate hemophilia from consideration. There is a particularly high rate of spontaneous mutation within the *FVIII* gene, and as a result, approximately 30% of newly diagnosed patients will have a negative family history of hemophilia.

In general, the severity of bleeding in hemophilia depends upon the percentage of residual, circulating clotting factor activity (Table 1.1). Patients with levels of >5–40% are classified as having mild hemophilia, those with levels of 1–5% as moderate, and those with less than 1% activity as having severe disease. The median age of diagnosis for someone with severe hemophilia is 1 month, compared to 8 months for those with moderate disease and 36 months for those with mild disease. Commonly, patients with severe disease will suffer from spontaneous bleeding, while those with mild-moderate disease typically bleed after trauma or surgery.

1 Management of an Infant with Hemophilia A

Table 1.1 Incidence of hemophilia A based upon the severity of disease

Severity	Factor level (%)	Incidence (%)
Mild	<1	20
Moderate	1–5	20
Severe	>5–40	60

Table 1.2 Spectrum of hemophilia A mutations and inhibitor incidence observed in patients with varying clinical severity

	Severe		Moderate		Mild	
Mutation type	Enrolled *n* (% of total)	Inhibitor *n* (% of mutation type)	Enrolled *n* (% of total)	Inhibitor *n* (% of mutation type)	Enrolled *n* (% of total)	Inhibitor *n* (% of mutation type)
Missense	100 (15)	9 (9)	106 (76)	11 (10)	175 (94)	13 (7)
Intron 22 inversion	283 (43)	102 (36)	6 (4)	1 (17)	1 (1)	
Frameshift	108 (16)	26 (24)	9 (6)	3 (33)		
Nonsense	79 (12)	21 (27)	2 (1)		1 (1)	
Splice site	19 (3)	8 (42)	6 (4)	1 (17)	5 (3)	
Large deletion	38 (6)	23 (61)	1 (1)			
Intron 1 inversion	10 (1)	4 (40)				
Small deletion	6 (1)				1 (1)	
Duplication	3 (1)	1 (33)	2 (1)			
None	15 (2)	4 (27)	7 (5)		4 (2)	
Total	661	198 (30)	139	16 (12)	187	13 (7)

Genetics

Many molecular defects have been described in the pathology of hemophilia A including large gene deletions, inversions, single gene rearrangements, deletions, and insertions (Table 1.2). Reported mutations leading to hemophilia A can be found at http://hadb.org.uk/ and https://www.cdc.gov/ncbddd/hemophilia/champs.html.

In our scenario, genetic testing is sent after the initial consultation and reveals a classic intron 22 inversion, which is the most common mutation seen in severe hemophilia A [5] (Fig. 1.3).

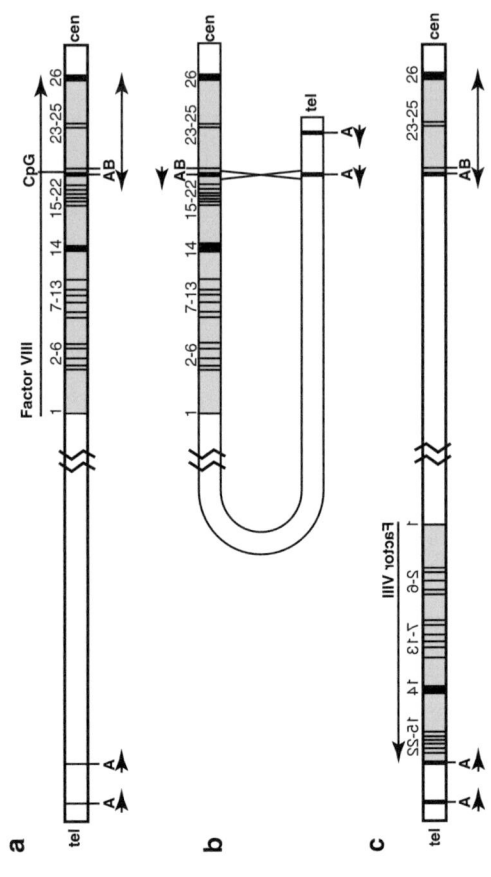

Fig. 1.3 Diagram of the factor VIII gene and illustration of the inversion model. (**a**) Region of Xq28 that includes the factor VIII gene, oriented with the telomere at the left, is depicted. Three copies of the A gene are indicated, two lying upstream of factor VIII and one inside intron 22. The location of the B transcript is also shown. The arrows indicate the direction of transcription of the factor VIII and internal A and B genes. The direction of the upstream A genes is hypothesized to be as shown. (**b**) Proposed homologous recombination between the intron 22 copy of gene A and one of the two upstream copies. A crossover between these two identical regions, oriented as shown, would result in an inversion of sequence between the two recombined A genes (**c**). A recombination could involve either of the upstream A genes, but only one is presented. The crossover could occur anywhere in the region of homology which includes the A genes. Reprinted with permission of Springer Nature. "Inversions disrupting the factor VIII gene are a common cause of severe haemophilia A", by Delia Lakich et al, 1993, Nature Genetics

Management of Newborns with Hemophilia

Factor Concentrates

The most common treatment of HA is FVIII replacement with intravenous FVIII concentrates. Concentrates are either plasma derived, containing varying amounts of VWF, or recombinant. Both undergo multiple viral and pathogen attenuation steps. No infectious complications have been reported in decades. Whether plasma derived or recombinant, the dose of factor delivery is calculated based upon the half-life of the product, the intravascular volume of distribution (on average 1 unit of FVIII per kilogram raises the plasma concentration by 2%), and the desired clotting factor activity.

Preferred products vary by hemophilia treatment center so discussion with a hemophilia specialist is advised. Additionally, the factor formulary in each hospital is managed by the blood bank or the pharmacy, and formulary influences concentrate selection, so inclusion of the blood bank or clinical pharmacy is recommended. Factor dosing in infants is challenging due to the vial size availability. For example, to raise the factor level of the 3 kg child in our clinical scenario to 50%, the dose should be 3 kg × 25 IU = 75 IU. However, the smallest available vial size of FVIII is 250 IU, so most clinicians would infuse the entire vial.

Antifibrinolytic Agents

Antifibrinolytic therapy to stabilize the fibrin clot is particularly useful in diminishing bleeding symptoms in locations with prominent fibrinolytic activity such as the mouth, gastrointestinal tract, and uterus [6]. These agents have a wide distribution and come in IV and oral forms. Case series suggest that they can be useful adjunctive agents in circumcision-related bleeding [7].

Comprehensive Care

A series of federally funded comprehensive hemophilia treatment centers (HTCs) exist to care for persons with hemophilia. They are typically staffed with hematologists, orthopedists, physical therapists, nurses, genetic counselors, psychologists, and social workers who specialize in the care of patients with bleeding disorders. It has been demonstrated that patients who receive their care in an HTC setting have improved outcomes and a longer life expectancy [8].

Clinical Pearls/Pitfalls
- Approximately 30% of persons with hemophilia A will have no known family history of bleeding disorders.
- Bleeding with circumcision is common in boys with hemophilia and should prompt a work-up in all cases.
- Laboratory evaluation is essential to establish the correct diagnosis, and communication with the special coagulation laboratory will facilitate expeditious results.
- Factor replacement is the preferred approach to bleeding; however, the type of product, plasma derived versus recombinant, continues to be debated due to the risk of inhibitor development.
- Communication with the blood bank or clinical pharmacy regarding available factor concentrates and vial sizes is important when dosing patients.
- Care of children with hemophilia requires consultation with a Hemophilia Treatment Center in order to obtain best patient outcomes.

References

1. Mannucci PM, Tuddenham EG. The hemophilias–from royal genes to gene therapy.[see comment][erratum appears in N Engl J Med. 2001;345(5):384]. [Review] [64 refs]. N Engl J Med 2001;344(23):1773–9.
2. Kulkarni R, Soucie JM, Lusher J, Presley R, Shapiro A, Gill J, et al. Sites of initial bleeding episodes, mode of delivery and age of diagnosis in babies with haemophilia diagnosed before the age of 2 years: a report from the Centers for Disease Control and Prevention's (CDC) Universal Data Collection (UDC) project. Haemophilia. 2009;15(6):1281–90.
3. Mansouritorghabeh H, Banihashem A, Modaresi A, Manavifar L. Circumcision in males with bleeding disorders. Mediterr J Hematol Infect Dis. 2013;5(1):e2013004.
4. Rodriguez V, Titapiwatanakun R, Moir C, Schmidt KA, Pruthi RK. To circumcise or not to circumcise? Circumcision in patients with bleeding disorders. Haemophilia. 2010;16(2):272–6.
5. Lakich D, Kazazian HH, Antonarakis SE, Gitschier J. Inversions disrupting the factor VIII gene are a common cause of severe haemophilia a. Nat Genet. 1993;5(3):236–41.
6. van Galen KPM, Engelen ET, Mauser-Bunschoten EP, van Es RJJ, Schutgens REG. Antifibrinolytic therapy for preventing oral bleeding in patients with haemophilia or Von Willebrand disease undergoing minor oral surgery or dental extractions. Cochrane Database Syst Rev. 2015;12:CD011385.
7. Yilmaz D, Akin M, Ay Y, Balkan C, ÇElik A, ErgÜN O, et al. A single centre experience in circumcision of haemophilia patients: Izmir protocol. Haemophilia. 2010;16(6):888–91.
8. Pipe SW, Kessler CM. Evidence-based guidelines support integrated disease management as the optimal model of haemophilia care. Haemophilia. 2016;22:3–5.

Clinical Care of a Child with Hemophilia A and Inhibitors

Surbhi Saini and Amy L. Dunn

Case Presentation You receive a call from the family of a 2-year-old boy with known severe hemophilia A (HA). He is on routine prophylaxis with recombinant factor VIII (rFVIII) concentrate once weekly and had his last dose yesterday. He has had 10 exposure days in total. The family reports that their son has a swollen right knee and is limping.

S. Saini
Department of Pediatrics, St. Louis Children's Hospital, St. Louis, MO, USA

Washington University in St. Louis School of Medicine, St. Louis, MO, USA

A. L. Dunn (✉)
Nationwide Children's Hospital, Division of Pediatric Hematology, Oncology and Bone Marrow Transplant, Columbus, OH, USA

Department of Pediatrics, The Ohio State University College of Medicine, Columbus, OH, USA
e-mail: amy.dunn@nationwidechildrens.org

Multiple-Choice Management Question

You suspect that this child may have developed an inhibitor to FVIII. Your next steps include:

A. Infuse factor VIII concentrate 50 IU/kg.
B. Inject emicizumab 3 mg/kg.
C. Perform a Bethesda assay.
D. **A and C**

Differential Diagnosis

The differential includes development of an inhibitor to FVIII, a breakthrough hemarthrosis without inhibitor formation, fracture, and non-bleeding-related soft tissue injuries.

Management

Fortunately, the patient lives close to the treatment center. After administering 50 IU/kg of rFVIII at home, the family presents to the hematology clinic. His knee is warm and has a palpable effusion but no physical findings of instability. His pain is well controlled with acetaminophen, ice, and a compression bandage. You suspect inhibitor formation. You call your coagulation lab and obtain a STAT Bethesda titer and FVIII level. The titer returns at 10 Bethesda units (BU), and the FVIII assay is <1%. This confirms presence of a high titer inhibitor.

Etiology of Inhibitor Development

Inhibitory alloantibodies to exogenous FVIII replacement concentrates, most commonly referred to as "inhibitors," occur in approximately 20–30% of patients with severe hemophilia A (HA). Inhibitor occurrence is less common in individuals with mild and moderate HA (2–3%). Inhibitors neutralize the exogenous

FVIII concentrate, rendering it ineffective and making it challenging to control bleeding complications. The majority of patients will develop inhibitors within the first 50 exposures to FVIII concentrate; a second peak in inhibitor occurrence is noted in late adulthood.

Genetic, environmental, and treatment-related factors play a role in inhibitor development [1]. Inhibitors are more common in individuals with large gene deletions and null mutations, than in individuals with missense mutations [2, 3]. Interestingly, patients with severe HA due to intron 22 inversion have a lower incidence of inhibitor development than other patients with severe HA. Inhibitor rates are also higher in patients with a family history of inhibitors and in African-Americans [4]. The cumulative incidence of inhibitors is higher in patients exposed to early, on-demand, intensive treatment regimens, and potentially in the setting of "danger signals" like large bleeds, tissue damage, inflammation, and surgery as opposed to early prophylactic regimens instituted in the absence of danger signals [5].

Since the introduction of recombinant FVIII concentrates, several studies have investigated the risk of inhibitors with the use of recombinant products versus Von Willebrand-containing plasma-derived FVIII (pdFVIII) concentrates [6, 7]. A recent randomized controlled trial to investigate the class effect of pdFVIII and rFVIII products found that pdFVIII were associated with a lower risk of inhibitor formation [8]. However, the generalizability and applicability of this study may be reduced by the limited racial and ethnic background of the study participants, majority use of on-demand treatment regimens, and lack of use of third-generation, and extended half-life rFVIII products.

Pathology

Mechanisms of inhibitor development are not completely understood. The immune response to FVIII involves factor uptake, processing, and presentation by the antigen-presenting cells to T-cells that lead to T-cell activation. Activated T-cells are involved in B-cell differentiation and eventual production of neutralizing antibodies by plasma cells. Immune modulatory genes specifically MHC class II, IL-10, TNF-α, and CTLA-4 influence this process, and variations of these gene products can influence the risk of inhibitor formation. These inhibitory antibodies are predominantly of the IgG4 and IgG1 subtype and are usually directed against the missing FVIII. Antibodies targeted against all domains of FVIII have been reported with A2 and C2 domains being the ones most frequently targeted [9, 10]. High titer inhibitors usually neutralize endogenous and exogenous FVIII completely, but a small subset of antibodies do not completely neutralize FVIII regardless of the titer and may be amenable to high-dose FVIII therapy.

Laboratory Findings

The antibody titer is measured with a Bethesda assay and is expressed in Bethesda units (BU). One Bethesda unit is the amount of antibody that decreases the plasma factor level by 50%, after incubation for 2 hours at 37 °C with normal plasma. The Centers for Disease Control and Prevention (CDC) and Nijmegen-Bethesda assay recommended modification of the Bethesda method increases the sensitivity of the method, although this is not widely adopted in all hemostasis laboratories (Fig. 2.1) [11].

Diagnosis

It is important to have a high index of suspicion for inhibitors in all patients with hemophilia, especially those with severe HA [12]. As opposed to patients with hemophilia B, where inhibitor occurrence might be associated with allergic or anaphylactoid reactions, patients with HA do not exhibit any overt physical signs or symptoms of inhibitor formation. The presence of an inhibitor should be suspected in any patient with hemophilia who does not respond to standard management of bleeding complications with factor concentrate replacement. Inhibitors should also be suspected in any patient who has increased breakthrough bleeding while on a weightappropriate dose of factor concentrate prophylaxis. As a matter of standard clinical practice, all patients on routine prophylaxis should be screened for the presence of inhibitors yearly.

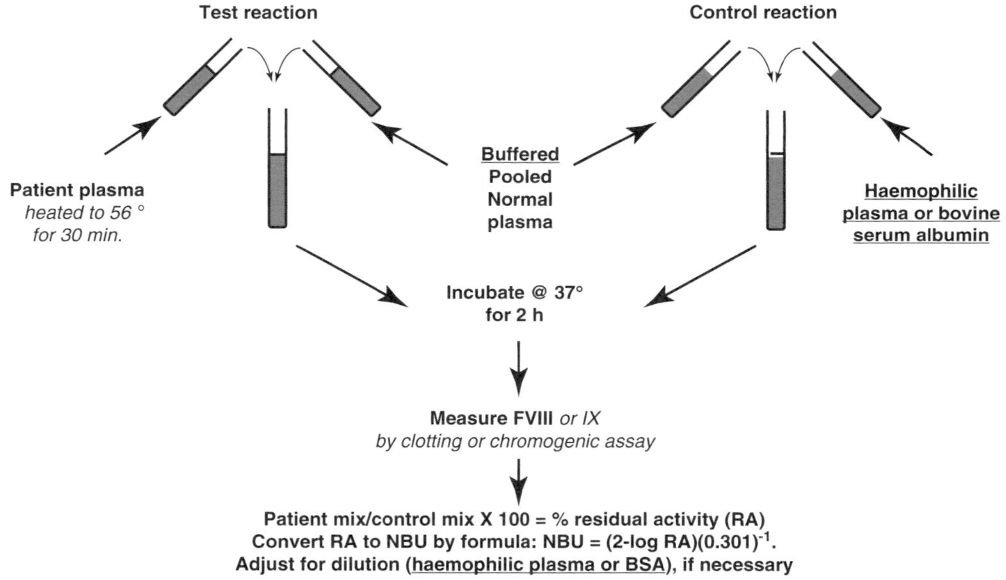

Fig. 2.1 Schematic of the CDC and Nijmegen-Bethesda assay based on the 1975 Bethesda assay with Nijmegen modifications underlined, and CDC-validated modifications in italics. (Used with permission. Miller CH. Laboratory testing for factor VIII and IX inhibitors in haemophilia: A review. *Haemophilia.* 2018;24(2):186–97)

Management

Inhibitor Eradication

Immune tolerance therapy (ITT) with repeated exposure to FVIII concentrate over a period of months to years may eradicate the antibody [13]. The success rate of ITT in patients with HA is approximately 80%. Both recombinant and VWF-containing products have been used successfully. Commonly accepted pre-ITT risk stratification for ITT success is described in Table 2.1.

Immune tolerance success is defined as a negative Bethesda assay, FVIII recovery of ≥66%, and FVIII half-life of ≥6 hours. ITT has been accomplished with both high-dose (100–200 IU/kg/day) and low-dose (50 IU/kg/three times per week) FVIII regimens. In the International Immune Tolerance Study, a randomized comparison of the high-dose FVIII (200 IU/kg/day) and low-dose FVIII (50 IU/kg three times a week) regimens, patients receiving high-dose FVIII achieved a negative inhibitor titer and normal FVIII recovery earlier than patients on the low-dose regimen, although the eventual success rate of ITT was not significantly different between the two groups. The rate of bleeding complications was higher for the low-dose group. Recent publications provide evidence that prompt start of ITT despite pre-ITT Bethesda titer may improve success rates [14, 15].

Immune modulatory therapy with the use of extracorporeal immune modulation, cyclophosphamide, and gammaglobulin was employed in the initial Malmö ITT regimens. More recently, a humanized monoclonal antibody to the B-cell CD20

Table 2.1 Patient characteristics that determine ITT success

	Good risk features	Poor risk features
Age at start of ITT	<8 years	≥8 years
Historical peak titer	<200 BU/mL	≥200 BU/mL
Pre-ITT titer	<10 BU/mL	≥10 BU/mL
Time to titer decline to <10 BU/mL before ITT	<24 months	≥24 months

antigen (rituximab) has been used for ITT in congenital hemophilia, and there is limited published data about outcomes. The use of immune modulators is generally reserved for patients where standard ITT with FVIII concentrates has been unsuccessful.

Intensive ITT regimens require adequate venous access which is challenging in young children. The use of central venous access devices is often necessary. The presence of these devices can lead to complications, particularly infectious, and can adversely impact the ITT outcomes.

Management of Acute Bleeding

Bleeding in the setting of a high titer inhibitor often requires bypassing therapy. The most commonly used bypassing agents include recombinant coagulation factor VIIa (FVIIa) [16] or activated prothrombin complex concentrate, FEIBA (factor VIII inhibitor bypassing activity) [17]. Both agents increase thrombin generation. These agents can be used to treat breakthrough bleeding but are also effective when used in a prophylactic manner to reduce bleeding frequency in patients with inhibitors. Please see Chap. 4 (hemophilia B and inhibitors) for a more detailed discussion of bypassing agents.

Future Therapies

Hemophilia care is changing rapidly, with the first nonfactor product approved for prophylactic use in persons with inhibitors in 2017. Emicizumab is a humanized, bispecific antibody that binds to FIXa and FX (Fig. 2.2) [18]. This essentially mimics the role of FVIII in the tenase complex and leads to FX activation and subsequent thrombin generation. This drug is approved for routine prophylaxis in patients with and without inhibitors. It is given subcutaneously in three different dosing strategies. All patients require four weekly loading doses of 3 mg/kg followed by maintenance therapy. The total monthly maintenance dose is 6 mg/kg and can be dosed as 1.5 mg/kg weekly, 3 mg/kg twice a month, or

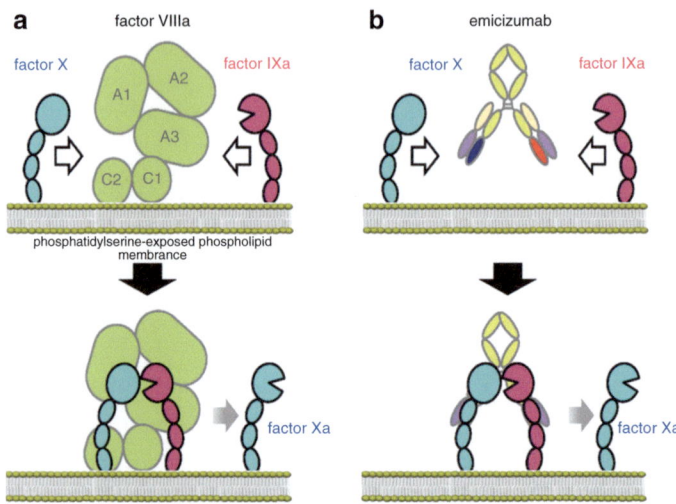

Fig. 2.2 Schematic illustrations of the action of FVIIIa and emicizumab as a cofactor promoting the interaction between FIXa and FX. (**a**) FVIIIa consists of the A1 subunit, the A2 subunit, and the light chain (A3, C1, and C2 subunits) and has multiple contacts with FIXaS2–S5, FXS6–S7, and the phosphatidylserine-exposed phospholipid membrane. Since FIXa and FX also have binding capability to phosphatidylserine-exposed phospholipid membrane, FVIIIa is considered to support the interaction between FIXa and FX on the membrane and to promote FIXa-catalyzed FX activation. (**b**) Emicizumab binding to FIXa and FX would promote the interaction between FIXa and FX on phosphatidylserine-exposed phospholipid membrane and exert FVIII-mimetic activity. The illustrations summarize the hypothesized mechanisms of action of emicizumab only and do not necessarily indicate precise molecular structures and positions. *FIXa* activated factor IX, *FVIII* factor VIII, *FVIIIa* activated factor VIII, *FX* factor X. (Used with permission. Shima M et al. Factor VIII–mimetic function of humanized bispecific antibody in Hemophilia A. *N Engl J Med.* 2016;374:2044–53)

6 mg/kg every 4 weeks. Acute breakthrough bleeding is managed with the use of activated factor VII (NovoSeven) in patients with inhibitors and FVIII concentrates in patients without inhibitors.

The most commonly reported adverse events are injection site reactions, headache, and arthralgia. However, thrombotic microangiopathy and thromboembolism have been reported. In all instances of TMA, these patients were treated with concomitant FEIBA >100 U/kg/24 hours. Given the long half-life of emicizumab, if the use of aPCCs is planned for a patient, emicizumab must be discontinued for a minimum of 6 months. Emicizumab interferes with multiple laboratory assays that are based on one-stage clotting assays such as the aPTT, one-stage FVIII activity, human Bethesda titer, and activated clotting time.

Concizumab is a humanized, monoclonal antibody against tissue factor pathway inhibitor (TFPI) that is administered subcutaneously. TFPI is a serine protease inhibitor that regulates coagulation via factor-Xa-dependent inhibition of factor VIIa. Attenuation of this inhibition has the potential to increase thrombin generation, hence restoring hemostasis. In the first human Phase 1 study of concizumab, no serious adverse events were noted [19]. In a subsequent dose-escalation study of concizumab, a dose-dependent increase in thrombin generation was noted. Currently, Phase 2 studies are underway to assess the ability of concizumab to decrease bleeding in patients with severe hemophilia A and B, with and without inhibitors.

Fitusiran is a small interfering RNA, coupled to N-acetylgalactosamine, that is administered subcutaneously and decreases antithrombin production. Antithrombin inactivates factor Xa and thrombin. Congenital deficiency of antithrombin causes hypercoagulability, and in murine HA studies, inhibition of antithrombin led to increased thrombin generation and decreased bleeding complications. Clinical Phase 1 and Phase 2 studies of monthly administration of fitusiran showed 70–90% reduction in antithrombin levels and overall decrease in bleeding events for patients with and without inhibitors [20]. Currently, Phase 3 studies of monthly dosing of fitusiran are underway.

Pearls
- Approximately 30% of patients with severe hemophilia A will develop inhibitory antibodies.
- Most inhibitors occur within the first 50 exposures to FVIII.

- Lack of clinical response to FVIII should prompt evaluation for inhibitors.
- Prophylaxis with bypassing agents is effective in persons with inhibitors.
- Immune tolerance therapy (ITT) is the gold standard for inhibitor eradication.
- Novel nonfactor therapeutics are rapidly changing the landscape of inhibitor management.

References

1. Oldenburg J, Brackmann HH, Schwaab R. Risk factors for inhibitor development in hemophilia A. Haematologica. 2000;85(10 Suppl):7–13; discussion – 4.
2. Schwaab R, Brackmann HH, Meyer C, Seehafer J, Kirchgesser M, Haack A, et al. Haemophilia A: mutation type determines risk of inhibitor formation. Thromb Haemost. 1995;74(6):1402–6.
3. Gouw SC, van den Berg HM, Oldenburg J, Astermark J, de Groot PG, Margaglione M, et al. F8 gene mutation type and inhibitor development in patients with severe hemophilia A: systematic review and meta-analysis. Blood. 2012;119(12):2922–34.
4. Astermark J, Berntorp E, White GC, Kroner BL, Group MS. The Malmö International Brother Study (MIBS): further support for genetic predisposition to inhibitor development in hemophilia patients. Haemophilia. 2001;7(3):267–72.
5. Gouw SC, van den Berg HM, Fischer K, Auerswald G, Carcao M, Chalmers E, et al. Intensity of factor VIII treatment and inhibitor development in children with severe hemophilia A: the RODIN study. Blood. 2013;121(20):4046–55.
6. Gouw SC, van der Bom JG, Auerswald G, Ettinghausen CE, Tedgård U, van den Berg HM. Recombinant versus plasma-derived factor VIII products and the development of inhibitors in previously untreated patients with severe hemophilia A: the CANAL cohort study. Blood. 2007;109(11):4693–7.
7. Gouw SC, van der Bom JG, Ljung R, Escuriola C, Cid AR, Claeyssens-Donadel S, et al. Factor VIII products and inhibitor development in severe hemophilia A. N Engl J Med. 2013;368(3):231–9.

8. Peyvandi F, Mannucci PM, Garagiola I, El-Beshlawy A, Elalfy M, Ramanan V, et al. A randomized trial of factor VIII and neutralizing antibodies in Hemophilia A. N Engl J Med. 2016;374(21):2054–64.
9. Meeks SL, Healey JF, Parker ET, Barrow RT, Lollar P. Nonclassical anti-C2 domain antibodies are present in patients with factor VIII inhibitors. Blood. 2008;112(4):1151–3.
10. Markovitz RC, Healey JF, Parker ET, Meeks SL, Lollar P. The diversity of the immune response to the A2 domain of human factor VIII. Blood. 2013;121(14):2785–95.
11. Miller CH. Laboratory testing for factor VIII and IX inhibitors in haemophilia: a review. Haemophilia. 2018;24(2):186–97.
12. Eckhardt CL, van Velzen AS, Peters M, Astermark J, Brons PP, Castaman G, et al. Factor VIII gene (F8) mutation and risk of inhibitor development in nonsevere hemophilia A. Blood. 2013;122(11):1954–62.
13. Hay CR, DiMichele DM, Study IIT. The principal results of the International Immune Tolerance Study: a randomized dose comparison. Blood. 2012;119(6):1335–44.
14. Eubanks J, Baldwin WH, Markovitz R, Parker ET, Cox C, Kempton CL, et al. A subset of high-titer anti-factor VIII A2 domain antibodies is responsive to treatment with factor VIII. Blood. 2016;127(16):2028–34.
15. Nakar C, Manco-Johnson MJ, Lail A, Donfield S, Maahs J, Chong Y, et al. Prompt immune tolerance induction at inhibitor diagnosis regardless of titre may increase overall success in haemophilia A complicated by inhibitors: experience of two U.S. centres. Haemophilia. 2015;21(3):365–73.
16. Konkle BA, Ebbesen LS, Erhardtsen E, Bianco RP, Lissitchkov T, Rusen L, et al. Randomized, prospective clinical trial of recombinant factor VIIa for secondary prophylaxis in hemophilia patients with inhibitors. J Thromb Haemost. 2007;5(9):1904–13.
17. Leissinger C, Gringeri A, Antmen B, Berntop E, Biasoli C, Carpenter S, et al. Anti-inhibitor coagulant complex prophylaxis in hemophilia with inhibitors. N Engl J Med. 2011;365(18):1684–92.
18. Oldenburg J, Mahlangu JN, Kim B, Schmitt C, Callaghan MU, Young G, et al. Emicizumab prophylaxis in Hemophilia A with inhibitors. N Engl J Med. 2017;377(9):809–18.
19. Chowdary P, Lethagen S, Friedrich U, Brand B, Hay C, Abdul Karim F, et al. Safety and pharmacokinetics of anti-TFPI antibody (concizumab) in healthy volunteers and patients with hemophilia: a randomized first human dose trial. J Thromb Haemost. 2015;13(5):743–54.
20. Pasi KJ, Rangarajan S, Georgiev P, Mant T, Creagh MD, Lissitchkov T, et al. Targeting of antithrombin in Hemophilia A or B with RNAi therapy. N Engl J Med. 2017;377(9):819–28.

Diagnosis and Management of a Patient with Newly Diagnosed Hemophilia B

Surbhi Saini and Amy L. Dunn

Case Presentation The emergency department requests consultation regarding a 6-year-old boy of Amish descent with no significant past medical history. He presented with right lower quadrant abdominal and right hip pain that started after he fell off his bicycle and hit the ground on his right side. His pain worsens with walking. On exam, the patient is unable to fully extend the right hip. His vital signs are stable, and his hemoglobin is 11 gm/dL. A diagnostic ultrasound reveals an iliopsoas hematoma.

S. Saini
Department of Pediatrics, St. Louis Children's Hospital, St. Louis, MO, USA

Washington University in St. Louis School of Medicine, St. Louis, MO, USA

A. L. Dunn (✉)
Nationwide Children's Hospital, Division of Pediatric Hematology, Oncology and Bone Marrow Transplant, Columbus, OH, USA

Department of Pediatrics, The Ohio State University College of Medicine, Columbus, OH, USA
e-mail: amy.dunn@nationwidechildrens.org

© Springer Nature Switzerland AG 2020
A. L. Dunn et al. (eds.), *Pediatric Bleeding Disorders*,
https://doi.org/10.1007/978-3-030-31661-7_3

Multiple-Choice Management Question

You suspect that this child has a congenital bleeding disorder. Do you:

A. Give a factor IX concentrate
B. Give cryoprecipitate
C. **Call for a STAT hematology consult**

Differential Diagnosis

The differential in this child includes congenital factor deficiencies, von Willebrand disease, hypo-/dysfibrinogenemia, thrombocytopenia, disseminated intravascular coagulation, liver disease, vitamin K deficiency, and severe platelet dysfunction.

Epidemiology

Hemophilia B (HB) is an X-linked recessive condition affecting approximately 1 in 20,000–25,000 male births. HB results from the congenital deficiency or absence of coagulation factor IX (FIX). There are approximately 4000 patients with HB in the United States, accounting for 15–20% of the hemophilia patient population. HB was formerly known as Christmas disease in honor of the first patient, Stephen Christmas, in whom the deficiency was first described. Certain populations including the Amish, and Mennonite communities have founder mutations within the HB gene, and due to large family sizes often have larger numbers of affected members. However, hemophilia A (HA) and von Willebrand disease are also present in the Amish community.

Pathophysiology

Coagulation FIX is a vitamin K-dependent serine protease that is synthesized in the liver. Factor IX is crucial for adequate thrombin generation and clot formation. Activated FIX complexes with activated factor VIII, and calcium on the phospholipid surface of platelets to form the tenase complex. This leads to generation of thrombin and, ultimately, a cross-linked fibrin clot (Fig. 3.1). Patients with HB cannot generate sufficient thrombin due to lack of FIX, and become dependent on the tissue factor (extrinsic) pathway. Circulating tissue factor pathway inhibitor (TFPI) downregulates the tissue factor pathway, making patients with hemophilia prone to excessive and prolonged bleeding.

Genetics

The FIX gene is 33 kilobases long and is located on the long arm of the X chromosome (Xq27.1). Multiple mutations are described in the FIX gene including small and large deletions and additions, rearrangements, and missense mutations (Fig. 3.2). A list of more than 1000 reported mutations can be found at the website https://www.cdc.gov/ncbddd/hemophilia/champs.html and http://www.factorix.org.

Clinical Presentation

The hallmark of HB-related bleeding is delayed bleeding, along with joint and muscle hemorrhages, and is indistinguishable from the bleeding diathesis noted in HA [1]. Patients with von Willebrand disease (VWD) more commonly experience mucocutaneous bleeding. As HB is X-linked, the vast majority of affected patients are male. Females can be affected in cases of extreme X chromosome lyonization or gene abnormalities such as Turner syndrome. It is increasingly recognized that female carriers of HB mutations can experience bleeding symptoms, and may have FIX levels that fall into the mild hemophilia range. Carrier females most commonly experience surgical and trauma-related bleeding as well as menorrhagia. Akin to patients with HA, the severity of bleeding in HB depends upon the percentage of residual, circulating clotting factor activity. Patients with levels of >5–40% are classified as having mild hemophilia, those

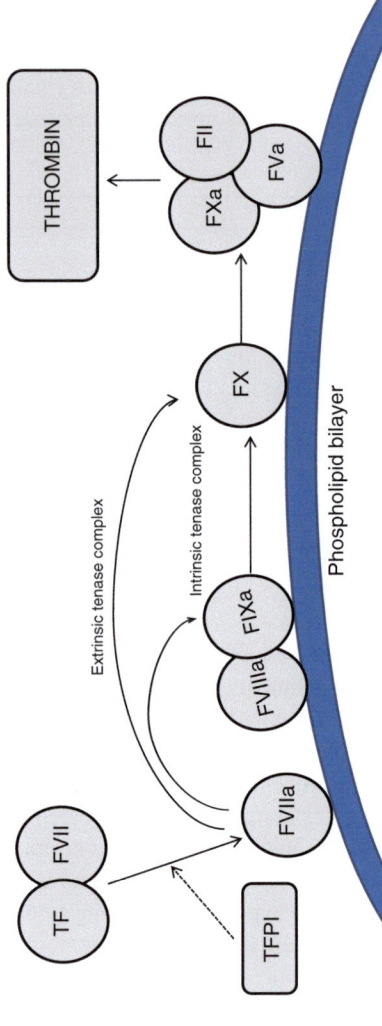

Fig. 3.1 Tenase complex. TF tissue factor, TFPI tissue factor pathway inhibitor, FVII factor VII, FVIIa activated factor VII, FVIIIa activated factor VIII, FIXa activated factor IX, FX factor X, FXa activated factor X, FII factor II (prothrombin), FVa activated factor V

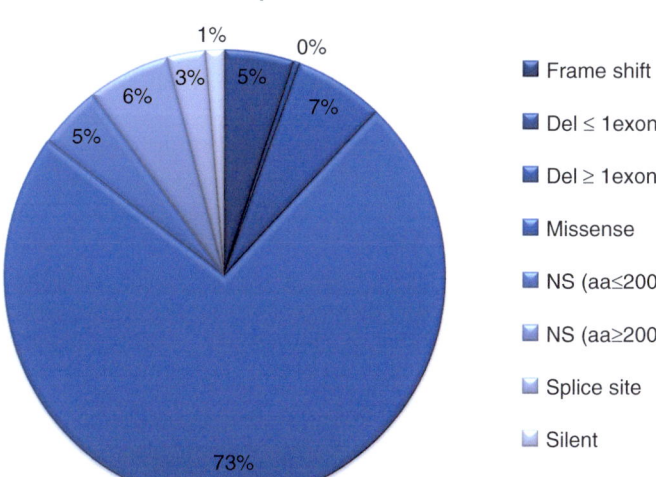

Fig. 3.2 Mutations reported in CHBMP

with levels of 1–5% as moderate, and those with less than 1% activity as having severe disease (see Chapter Hemophilia A without inhibitors).

Diagnosis

Hemophilia B is usually associated with a prolonged aPTT, and is confirmed by a low FIX level and a genetic mutation in the FIX gene (see Chapter Hemophilia A without inhibitors for details).

Management

Fresh frozen plasma has minimal amounts of FIX and is not sufficient for treatment of patients with HB. Cryoprecipitate does not contain FIX and is not indicated in HB. Desmopressin is also not indicated for treatment of HB. The mainstay of treatment is infusion of a FIX concentrate. The dose and frequency of factor administration are calculated based upon the pharmacokinetics of each particular product and the desired plasma concentration. One international unit (IU) of FIX per kilogram of body weight raises the FIX plasma concentration by about 1%. For example, to raise the factor level of a 30 kg child with severe HB to 100%, the dose should be 30 kg × 100 IU = 3000 IU. Forty percent activity is considered hemostatic in most cases; however, in the setting of surgery or life-/limb-threatening hemorrhage, higher levels are necessary (Table 3.1). Factor replacement is typically provided in two settings: "on-demand" treatment used for the acute management of bleeding episodes or "prophylaxis" therapy typically administered on a regular basis to prevent long-term complications of degenerative joint disease [2].

Table 3.1 Suggested approaches to treatment of bleeding episodes using standard half-life concentrates

Bleed site	Desired activity	Length of therapy	Ancillary measures to consider
Central nervous system	100%	7–14 days then strongly consider prophylactic therapy for a minimum of 6 months	Continuous infusion FIX; anti-epileptic prophylaxis; surgical intervention
Persistent oral/mucosal	30–60%	3–7 days	Antifibrinolytic therapy; custom mouthpiece
Retropharyngeal	80–100%	7–14 days	Continuous infusion FIX; antifibrinolytic therapy
Nose	30–60%	1–3 days	Packing, cautery; saline spray/gel; vasoconstrictor spray; antifibrinolytic therapy
Gastrointestinal	40–80%	3–7 days	Antifibrinolytic therapy; endoscopy with cautery

Table 3.1 (continued)

Bleed site	Desired activity	Length of therapy	Ancillary measures to consider
Persistent gross urinary	40–60%	1–3 days	Vigorous hydration; evaluation for stones/urinary tract infection; avoid antifibrinolytic therapy; glucocorticoids
Muscle	40–80%	Every third day until pain-free movement	Rest, ice, compression, elevation; physical therapy
Iliopsoas	80–100%	Until radiographic evidence of resolution	Continuous infusion FIX; bed rest; physical therapy
Joint	40–80%	1–2 days	Rest, ice, compression, elevation; physical therapy
Target joint	80% day 1, 40% day 3	3–4 days	Rest, ice, compression, elevation; physical therapy

Factor IX concentrates manufactured using pooled human plasma ("plasma derived") have been infrequently used in the United States since the introduction of recombinant FIX products in the late 1990s. Most recently, bioengineered FIX concentrates with extended half-lives have become available [3]. These products have a three- to fivefold increase in half-life vis-à-vis standard FIX concentrates and allow for decreased dosing frequency. Several mechanisms have been employed for this increase in half-life including coupling to neonatal Fc receptors (rFIXFc), polyethylene glycol (PEGylated FIX), or albumin (rFIX-FP).

Complications

Hemophilia B is rarely complicated by the development of inhibitory antibodies (see chapter on HB inhibitors). While these antibodies occur in only approximately 3% of patients with severe

HB, they are often accompanied by anaphylactoid reactions to exogenous FIX which can be life-threatening [4].

Bleeding into the ankles, knees, and elbows is a hallmark of HB, and the resultant arthropathy is the leading cause of morbidity for patients with HB. Arthropathy leads to missed school, work, chronic pain, and decreased quality of life. The mechanisms of blood induced joint damage are incompletely understood, but free radical formation driven by free iron and inflammatory cytokines from white blood cells likely triggers many of the degenerative changes. Changes include hypertrophic synovitis, cartilage derangements, and bone issues including osteopenia and cyst formation.

Future Therapies

The concept of "rebalancing hemostasis" and thus increasing thrombin generation has been applied to the development of another category of products to treat hemophilia. Fitusiran (ALN-AT3SC), a small interfering RNA that decreases natural antithrombin levels, is currently undergoing an open-label extension trial. Concizumab (monoclonal anti-TFPI antibody) inhibits TFPI leading to increase in thrombin generation via the TF-FVIIa pathway. Preliminary clinical trials are being conducted.

Gene therapy is a promising new frontier for patients with HB. Gene therapy using adeno-associated viral vectors (AAV) is well into late phase clinical trials for patients with HB. The initial cohort of adult HB patients who underwent gene therapy with the AAV vectors have demonstrated sustained, elevated plasma FIX activity levels for well over 7 years [5].

Our Patient's Case You respond to the ED immediately and learn that there is a strong family history of hemophilia B in this child. In addition, his PTT is elevated. The FIX level is pending. Because iliopsoas bleeds can lead to long-term neuromuscular damage, you recommend administration of FIX concentrate to raise FIX levels to 80–100%, with plans to keep trough levels

>50% for 7 days. You also recommend admission and bed rest. You tell the family that treatment for this type of bleed usually lasts about 2–6 weeks, and then, a slow return to activities and physical therapy is advised due to the risk of rebleeding.

> **Clinical Pearls**
> - Hemophilia B accounts for approximately 20% of all cases of hemophilia.
> - Certain communities including the Amish and Mennonites have large populations affected by hemophilia B.
> - Hemophilia B was formerly known as Christmas disease.
> - Fresh frozen plasma, cryoprecipitate, and DDAVP are not affective treatments for hemophilia B.

References

1. Clausen N, Petrini P, Claeyssens-Donadel S, Gouw SC, Liesner R, Group PaRoDoIdRS. Similar bleeding phenotype in young children with haemophilia A or B: a cohort study. Haemophilia. 2014;20(6):747–55.
2. Ullman M, Zhang QC, Grosse SD, Recht M, Soucie JM, Investigators HTCN. Prophylaxis use among males with haemophilia B in the United States. Haemophilia. 2017;23(6):910–7.
3. Iorio A, Fischer K, Blanchette V, Rangarajan S, Young G, Morfini M, et al. Tailoring treatment of haemophilia B: accounting for the distribution and clearance of standard and extended half-life FIX concentrates. Thromb Haemost. 2017;117(6):1023–30.
4. Puetz J, Soucie JM, Kempton CL, Monahan PE, Investigators HTCNH. Prevalent inhibitors in haemophilia B subjects enrolled in the Universal Data Collection database. Haemophilia. 2014;20(1):25–31.
5. Nathwani AC, Reiss UM, Tuddenham EG, Rosales C, Chowdary P, McIntosh J, et al. Long-term safety and efficacy of factor IX gene therapy in hemophilia B. N Engl J Med. 2014;371(21):1994–2004.

Approach to a Child with Hemophilia B and Anaphylaxis to Factor IX

Surbhi Saini and Amy L. Dunn

Case Presentation You are urgently called to the infusion clinic after a 2-year-old male with a known history of severe hemophilia B (HB) develops facial swelling and hives with itching shortly after being given an infusion of clotting factor IX (FIX) concentrate to treat a knee hemarthrosis. As you are examining him, he starts coughing and develops difficulty breathing. He has tachycardia and tachypnea. His mother reports that this is his third infusion of FIX concentrate.

S. Saini
Department of Pediatrics, St. Louis Children's Hospital, St. Louis, MO, USA

Washington University in St. Louis School of Medicine, St. Louis, MO, USA

A. L. Dunn (✉)
Nationwide Children's Hospital, Division of Pediatric Hematology, Oncology and Bone Marrow Transplant, Columbus, OH, USA

Department of Pediatrics, The Ohio State University College of Medicine, Columbus, OH, USA
e-mail: amy.dunn@nationwidechildrens.org

Multiple-Choice Management Question

After immediate cardiopulmonary stabilization that included intravenous steroids, diphenhydramine, and intramuscular epinephrine, your patient's allergic symptoms are resolving. He is admitted to the hospital for careful observation. Your next steps in medical management will include:

1. Urinalysis to evaluate for proteinuria
2. Bethesda assay for factor IX inhibitors
3. Avoidance of factor IX
4. **All of the above**

Differential Diagnosis

The differential diagnosis in this toddler with an allergic reaction to FIX-containing concentrate includes the emergence of inhibitors to FIX as well as latex allergies.

Laboratory Findings

Laboratory evaluation of this patient can help in making a confirmatory diagnosis. An elevated partial thromboplastin time (PTT) and decreased plasma FIX activity assay confirm the diagnosis of HB. Persistent prolongation of the PTT after a 1:1 mix of the patient's plasma with pooled normal plasma (mixing study or inhibitor screen) indicates the presence of an inhibitor to FIX. The presence of a FIX inhibitor can be confirmed by the Bethesda assay, which gives a numerical value to the concentration of the coagulation factor inhibitor present in plasma. One Bethesda unit (BU) is defined as the amount of inhibitor in the test (patient) plasma that can neutralize 50% of the coagulation factor activity of normal pooled plasma after incubation for 2 hours at 37 °Celsius. The Nijmegen modification, which includes standardization of pH and protein concentration, has greater sensitivity and specificity and is the gold standard for inhibitor testing per the International Society on Thrombosis and Hemostasis (ISTH) [1].

Clinical Characteristics and Risk Factors

Hemophilia B (HB) is a rare condition, occurring in approximately 1:20–25,000 live male births. Patients with HB have a complete absence or deficiency of coagulation FIX. Clinically, HB is classified based upon the residual plasma FIX activity as mild (>5–40%), moderate (1–5%), and severe (<1%). Standard treatment approaches involve regular or episodic replacement with exogenous FIX-containing concentrates, which can be recombinant or plasma derived.

Over the last two decades, FIX-containing concentrates have been increasingly available, with an enhanced safety profile, and improved pharmacokinetics. Consequently, the development of FIX inhibitors has emerged as one of the most serious complications of HB treatment. Inhibitors are alloantibodies that neutralize exogenous factor concentrates, making it difficult to achieve hemostasis in such patients.

Inhibitor development in HB is exceedingly rare, occurring in approximately 1–6% of the patients with HB [2]. This is in contrast to hemophilia A (HA), where approximately 25–30% of the patients with severe disease will develop inhibitors [3]. This discrepancy has been attributed to several nongenetic factors, which include (i) structural analogy of FIX to other serine proteases that may confer some tolerance, (ii) smaller size and fewer immunologically active epitopes on the FIX protein, and (iii) higher extravascular distribution of FIX as compared to factor VIII.

The rarity of inhibitors in HB limits our understanding of its pathophysiology and an understanding of host and treatment-related risk factors. One of the largest registries of patients with FIX inhibitors, under the auspices of the ISTH, included 94 patients from around the world. The median age at detection of the inhibitor was 19.5 months (range 9–156 months), and the median number of exposure days to FIX was 11 days (range

2–180 days). While the racial and ethnic background of patients has been shown to influence inhibitor formation in HA, no such correlation has been established for HB. Inhibitors in HB generally occur in patients with severe deficiency, and it is extremely rare for patients with mild/moderate deficiency to develop inhibitors. An antibody titer of ≥ 5 Bethesda units, defined as a high-responding inhibitor, occurs in the majority of persons with HB that develop inhibitors. Strong anamnestic responses are also common, with reappearance of inhibitor on re-exposure to FIX.

Genetic risk factors and family history play a significant role in determining the risk for inhibitor formation in HB [4, 5]. A recent analysis of the Centers for Disease Control and Prevention's Hemophilia B Mutation Database (CHBMP) revealed 249 patients with HB for whom genetic mutations and inhibitor status were available (Fig. 4.1) [6]. Missense mutations were identified in the majority of the patients (67%); however, the occurrence of inhibitors was significantly higher in those with null mutations (nonsense mutations, large deletions, and frameshift mutations). Moreover, inhibitor incidence was higher in patients with deletions more than 50 base pairs, and those where a nonsense mutation led to early termination of protein synthesis. This strongly suggests that a complete or near-complete lack of endogenous FIX protein increases the risk of inhibitor formation. It has been postulated that patients with detectable FIX protein develop central tolerance to the "self"-protein and are protected from inhibitor formation upon exposure to exogenous FIX.

The simultaneous occurrence of severe allergic or anaphylactic reactions with the appearance of inhibitors is unique to HB. In the ISTH registry, approximately 60% of the patients that developed inhibitors presented with severe allergic or anaphylactic reactions [7]. Symptoms ranged from itchy, erythematous rashes to bronchospasm and severe hypotension. These reactions are variable in severity and can start off mildly with a rash and cough but progress rapidly to syncope and vascular collapse. Patients from families where other members have had severe allergic reactions to FIX are particularly susceptible. Several studies have sought to investigate an Ig-E-mediated mechanism for the allergic reactions

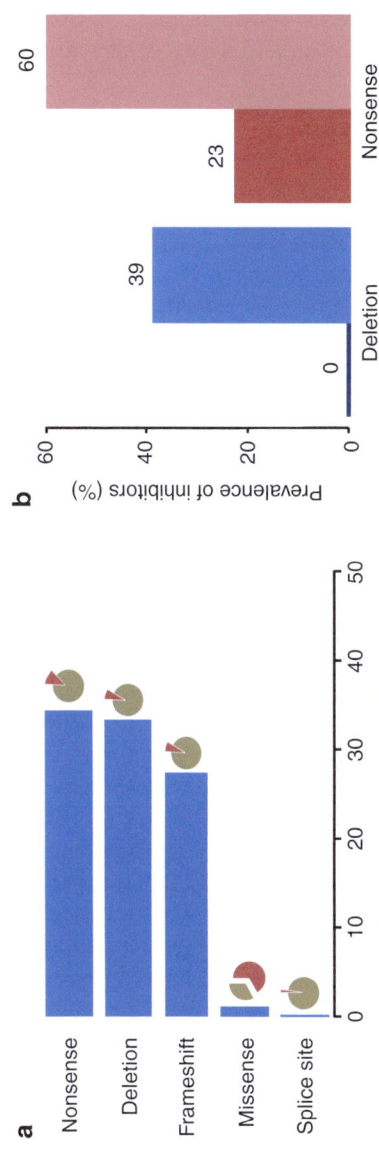

Fig. 4.1 (**a**) Data in the CHBMP database were used to determine the prevalence of inhibitors in different classes of mutations in the *F9* gene ($N = 249$). The pie chart alongside each bar depicts the fraction of patients (dark segment) who carried that particular class of mutation. (**b**) Patients with deletions and nonsense mutations were further divided into two groups. Prevalence of inhibitors was determined in patients where the deletion in the *F9* gene was less than 50 (open bar) or greater than 50 (grey, filled bar) base pairs. Similarly, patients with the nonsense mutations were classified into those where the mutation resulted in FIX protein truncated within the first 100 amino acids (unfilled bar) or thereafter (filled, grey bar)

noted in HB, but to date, this has not been decisively established. For the same reason, the term "anaphylactoid" reactions rather than anaphylactic reactions is preferred by some practitioners.

Management

The presence of FIX inhibitors neutralizes the hemostatic functions of infused FIX concentrates, thus making the management of bleeding in these patients extremely challenging. In clinical practice, the goals of management for patients with FIX inhibitors are (i) prevention and treatment of bleeding complications and (ii) eradication of the FIX inhibitor.

Prevention and Treatment of Bleeding Complications

High-Responding Inhibitors

The majority of patients with HB who develop inhibitors form high-responding (≥ 5 BU) inhibitors with or without an allergic reaction. The mainstay of therapeutic approach to treating and preventing bleeding episodes in patients with high-responding FIX inhibitors involves strategies that bypass the requirement of FIX for thrombin generation. The agents used are together known as "bypassing agents." Currently, the two agents that are most commonly used are recombinant coagulation factor VIIa (FVIIa) (rFVIIa; NovoSeven RT®) and activated prothrombin complex concentrate (aPCC; FEIBA®) (Table 4.1). In a prospective, randomized, crossover comparison of clinical equivalency between rFVIIa and aPCC in the treatment of joint hemorrhages, both agents showed similar hemostatic efficacy (~80%). Interestingly, 30–40% of the patients in the study reported greater subjective satisfaction with one product over the other, distributed equally between rFVIIa and aPCC.

Both treatment strategies are complicated by the need of reliable venous access. There is a risk of arterial and venous thromboembolism and/or disseminated intravascular thrombosis with

4 Hemophilia B and Anaphylaxis

Table 4.1 Comparison of the key characteristics of hemostatic bypassing agents recombinant coasulation factor VIIa (FVIIa) (rFVIIa; NovoSeven RT®) and activated prothrombin complex concentrate (aPCC; FEIBA®)

	rFVIIa	aPCC
Active components	Recombinant coasulation factor VIIa (FVIIa)	Plasma-derived factors II, IX, XI, and VIIa
Half-life (hours)	2–3	8–12
Treatment of acute bleeding	270 ug/kg × 1 or 90–120 ug/kg every 2 hours until hemostasis achieved	50–100 IU/kg every 8–12 hours until hemostasis achieved
Prophylaxis schedule	90–270 ug/kg once daily	75–100 IU/kg three times a week
Advantages	Low infusion volumes Factor IX free – no risk of anamnesis No risk of transmission of blood-borne infections	Less frequent dosing Less expensive
Disadvantages	Requires frequent dosing More expensive	Larger infusion volumes Contains factor IX; contraindicated in patients with factor IX inhibitors at risk of anaphylaxis Risk of transmission of blood-borne infections

rFVIIa and aPCC, higher with aPCC. More importantly, the hemostatic efficacy of both rFVIIa and aPCC is inferior to factor replacement in patients without inhibitors, resulting in more breakthrough bleeding episodes. In addition, there are no established biomarkers or laboratory tests that can help guide therapeutic dosing and efficacy with the use of rFVIIa or aPCC.

In patients with FIX inhibitors, especially those that manifest an allergic phenotype, rFVIIa is frequently chosen as the first line of bypassing therapy to minimize re-exposure to FIX and the risk of anaphylaxis and anamnesis. rFVIIa is used for the prevention (prophylaxis) and on-demand treatment of bleeding, as well as perioperatively for surgical hemostasis. For acute bleeding episodes, dosing regimens most often employed use 90–120 ug/kg of rFVIIa given every 2–3 hours until hemostasis is achieved. Alternatively, a single large dose of 270 ug/kg given once has been shown to be effective in achieving hemostasis and relieving pain associated with bleeding (e.g., hemarthrosis), without additional risk of thrombosis. For prophylaxis, rFVIIa is often used in doses ranging from 90 to 270 ug/kg once daily. It is to be noted that rFVIIa is available in vial sizes of 1 mg, 2 mg, 5 mg, and 8 mg only. It is recommended that doses for each patient be rounded off to the nearest vial size, so as to use the entire contents of the vial and avoid wastage.

Low-Responding Inhibitors

A minority of patients with FIX inhibitors have low-responding inhibitors (persistent levels of <5BU despite repeated exposure) without any allergic reactions. In such patients, treatment of hemorrhagic episodes can be carried out with higher than standard doses of FIX concentrate. Doses are calculated to overcome the inhibitor titer and allow a hemostatic level of FIX. In such patients, pharmacokinetic studies to document FIX recovery and half-life in the non-bleeding state can help guide therapy in the event of a bleeding complication.

Eradication of Factor IX Inhibitors

Despite the use of as-needed or daily prophylactic bypassing agents, patients with inhibitors struggle with frequent breakthrough bleeding, progressive joint damage, and decline in health-related quality of life compared to patients without inhibitors. Inhibitor eradication in HA and HB, termed immune tolerance induction (ITI), is a treatment strategy where repeated, frequent exposure to factor VIII or IX downregulates the established antibody response and induces a state of immune tolerance to factor VIII or IX.

Owing to higher event frequency of inhibitors in HA, a large part of the scientific body of literature regarding ITI relates to

HA. Experiences with ITI in HB are limited to small case series or case reports (Table 4.2). In addition, the reported success rate of achieving tolerance in HB has been widely variable [8]. Early experiences utilizing the Malmö protocol reported successful tolerance induction in six of the seven (85%) patients, with one patient eventually losing tolerance with successful re-induction. The Malmö protocol employed high doses of FIX concentrate with immune modulation (cyclophosphamide, intravenous IgG) with or without adsorption of antibodies to protein A. Subsequently, the North American Immune Tolerance Registry (NAITR) and the International Registry of Factor IX Inhibitors reported an overall 14–31% success rate in HB ITI [7, 9]. High-risk features for ITI failure in the NAITR cohorts were high-responding inhibitors, historical peak titer ≥ 50 BU, pre-induction titer of ≥ 10 BU, allergic phenotype, and ≥ 47 months lag between inhibitor detection and initiation of ITI.

The presence of allergic and/or anaphylactic reactions in patients with FIX inhibitors requires desensitization to FIX in order to initiate high-dose FIX ITI. A desensitization protocol most commonly adopted was first described by Dioun in 1998 where escalating doses of FIX were administered intravenously under careful monitoring. Furthermore, given the poor outcomes with ITI in HB, adjunctive immunomodulatory strategies employing rituximab, mycophenolate mofetil, dexamethasone, and intravenous immunoglobulins have been used with variable success (Table 4.2).

The development of nephrotic syndrome is a unique complication of ITI in HB [22, 23]. This occurs more commonly in patients who present with allergic/anaphylactoid reactions and presents 6–9 months after ITI initiation. Patients present with proteinuria, edema, and hypoalbuminemia, much like idiopathic nephrotic syndrome. However, ITI-related nephrotic syndrome is most commonly steroid resistant and requires complete withdrawal of exposure to FIX.

Table 4.2 Immune tolerance strategies in patients with hemophilia B and inhibitors

Publication	Age	Highest inhibitor	Allergic reactions	Regimen	Response
Dioun (1998) [10]	14 months	67.5 BU	Y	Desensitization to escalating doses of FIX	Successful
	9 years	51 BU	Y	Desensitization to escalating doses of FIX	Successful
Shibata (2003) [11]	4 years	3 BU	Y	Desensitization to escalating doses of FIX, hydrocortisone	Failure with development of nephrotic syndrome 10 months into ITI
	6 years	11 BU	Y		Successful
	1 year	1.8 BU	Y		Successful
Mathias (2004) [12]	11 years	70 BU	N	High-dose recombinant FIX, rituximab	Failure with reemergence of inhibitor within 3 months of ITI
Fox (2006) [13]	17 years	39 BU	Y	High-dose plasma-derived FIX, rituximab	Initial complete response with reemergence of the inhibitor at 10 months and development of nephrotic syndrome at 12 months
Curry (2007) [14]	3.5 years	10.3 BU	Y	Desensitization to escalating doses of recombinant FIX and hydrocortisone followed by the Malmö protocol (IVIG, cyclophosphamide, high-dose recombinant FIX)	Complete response within 6 weeks

Alexander (2008) [15]	8 years	1.6 BU	Y	Desensitization to escalating doses of plasma-derived FIX, rituximab	Complete response within 6 weeks; worsening FIX kinetics at 13 months that required another course of ITI with same agents
Chuansumrit (2008) [16]	10 years	70 BU	Y	Desensitization to escalating doses of plasma-derived FIX, rituximab	Partial response with reduction in inhibitor titer
Klarmann (2008) [17]	14 months	4.8 BU	Y	MMF, dexamethasone, IVIG, high-dose plasma-derived FIX	Partial response within 21 months
	5.5 years	7 BU	N		Complete response within 24 months
Beutel (2009) [18]	11.5 years	6.2 BU	Y	Rituximab, MMF, dexamethasone, IVIG, and high-dose FIX	Complete response within 2 months
Barnes (2010) [19]	10 years	1 BU	Y	High-dose plasma-derived FIX, rituximab	Complete response within 1 month
Holstein (2014) [20]	11 years	2.6 BU	Y	High-dose FIX, dexamethasone, rituximab, MMF, and IVIG	Sustained response for 7 years after which ITI with same agents was repeated with success
Bon (2015) [21]	2 years	25 BU	Y	Desensitization to escalating doses of FIX	Partial response with detectable inhibitor titer

Clinical Pearls and Pitfalls
- Inhibitor development in patients with hemophilia B is a rare but significant complication.
- FIX inhibitors are most common in patients with severe disease caused by large deletions or frameshift mutations and occur early in life.
- Allergic or anaphylactic reactions to FIX concentrate infusions may precede or coincide with inhibitor detection in HB. It is recommended that all patients with severe HB and high-risk mutations receive their first 20–25 infusions of FIX concentrate under medical supervision.
- Bleeding episodes can be treated or prevented with the use of bypassing agents in patients with FIX inhibitors, albeit with moderate success.
- Immune tolerance induction using high-dose FIX and immune modulating agents has been used with variable success in eradicating FIX inhibitors.
- The development of steroid-resistant nephrotic syndrome can complicate ITI in HB, requiring complete cessation of further FIX exposure.

References

1. Miller CH, Platt SJ, Rice AS, Kelly F, Soucie JM. Validation of Nijmegen-Bethesda assay modifications to allow inhibitor measurement during replacement therapy and facilitate inhibitor surveillance. J Thromb Haemost. 2012;10(6):1055–61.
2. Barnes C, Davis A, Furmedge J, Egan B, Donnan L, Monagle P. Induction of immune tolerance using rituximab in a child with severe haemophilia B with inhibitors and anaphylaxis to factor IX. Haemophilia. 2010;16(5):840–1.
3. Darby SC, Keeling DM, Spooner RJD, Wan Kan S, Giangrande PLF, Collins PW, Hill FGH, Hay CRM. The incidence of factor VIII and factor IX inhibitors in the hemophilia population of the UK and their effect on subsequent mortality, 1977-99. J Thromb Haemost. 2004;2(7):1047–54.

4. Ljung R, Petrini P, Tengborn L, Sjorin E. Haemophilia B mutations in Sweden: a population-based study of mutational heterogeneity. Br J Haematol. 2001;113(1):81–6.
5. Puetz J, Soucie JM, Kempton CL, Monahan PE. Prevalent inhibitors in haemophilia B subjects enrolled in the Universal Data Collection database. Haemophilia. 2014;20(1):25–31.
6. Saini S, Hamasaki-Katagiri N, Pandey GS, Yanover C, Guelcher C, Simhadri VL, Dandekar S, Guerrera MF, Kimchi-Sarfaty C, Sauna ZE. Genetic determinants of immunogenicity to factor IX during the treatment of haemophilia B. Haemophilia. 2015;21(2):210–8.
7. Chitlur M, Warrier I, Rajpurkar M, Lusher JM. Inhibitors in factor IX deficiency a report of the ISTH-SSC international FIX inhibitor registry (1997-2006). Haemophilia. 2009;15(5):1027–31.
8. Hay CR, DiMichele DM. The principal results of the International Immune Tolerance Study: a randomized dose comparison. Blood. 2012;119(6):1335–44.
9. DiMichele DM, Kroner BL. Analysis of the North American Immune Tolerance Registry (NAITR) 1993–1997: current practice implications. Vox Sang. 1999;77(Suppl. 1):31–2.
10. Dioun AF, Ewenstein BM, Geha RS, Schneider LC. IgE-mediated allergy and desensitization to factor IX in hemophilia B. J Allergy Clin Immunol. 1998;102(1):113–7.
11. Shibata M, Shima M, Misu H, Okimoto Y, Giddings JC, Yoshioka A. Management of haemophilia B inhibitor patients with anaphylactic reactions to FIX concentrates. Haemophilia. 2003;9(3):269–71.
12. Mathias M, Khair K, Hann I, Liesner R. Rituximab in the treatment of alloimmune factor VIII and IX antibodies in two children with severe haemophilia. Br J Haematol. 2004;125(3):366–8.
13. Fox RA, Neufeld EJ, Bennett CM. Rituximab for adolescents with haemophilia and high titre inhibitors. Haemophilia. 2006;12(3):218–22.
14. Curry NS, Misbah SA, Giangrande PLF, Keeling DM. Achievement of immune tolerance in a patient with haemophilia B and inhibitory antibodies, complicated by an anaphylactoid reaction. Haemophilia. 2007;13(3):328–30.
15. Alexander S, Hopewell S, Hunter S, Chouksey A. Rituximab and desensitization for a patient with severe factor IX deficiency, inhibitors, and history of anaphylaxis. J Pediatr Hematol Oncol. 2008;30(1):93–5.
16. Chuansumrit A, Moonsup Y, Sirachainan N, Benjaponpitak S, Suebsangad A, Wongwerawattanakoon P. The use of rituximab as an adjuvant for immune tolerance therapy in a hemophilia B boy with inhibitor and anaphylaxis to factor IX concentrate. Blood Coagul Fibrinolysis. 2008;19(3):208–11.
17. Klarmann D, Martinez Saguer I, Funk MB, Knoefler R, von Hentig N, Heller C, Kreuz W. Immune tolerance induction with mycophenolatemofetil in two children with haemophilia B and inhibitor. Haemophilia. 2008;14(1):44–9.

18. Beutel K, Hauch H, Rischewski J, Kordes U, Schneppenheim J, Schneppenheim R. ITI with high-dose FIX and combined immunosuppressive therapy in a patient with severe haemophilia B and inhibitor. Hamostaseologie. 2009;29(2):155–7.
19. Barnes C, Davis A, Furmedge J, Egan B, Donnan L, Monagle P. Induction of immune tolerance using rituximab in a child with severe haemophilia B with inhibitors and anaphylaxis to factor IX. Haemophilia. 2010;16(5):840–1.
20. Holstein K, Schneppenheim R, Schrum J, Bokemeyer C, Langer F. Successful second ITI with factor IX and combined immunosuppressive therapy. Hamostaseologie. 2017;34(Suppl 1):S5–8.
21. Bon A, Morfini M, Dini A, Mori F, Barni S, Gianluca S, de Martino M, Novembre E. Desensitization and immune tolerance induction in children with severe factor IX deficiency; inhibitors and adverse reactions to replacement therapy: a case-report and literature review. Ital J Pediatr. 2015;41:12.
22. Dharnidharka VR, Takemoto C, Ewenstein BM, Seymour R, William Harris H. Membranous glomerulonephritis and nephrosis post factor IX infusions in hemophilia B. Pediatr Nephrol. 1998;12(8):654–7.
23. Ewenstein BM, Takemoto C, Warrier I, Lusher J, Saidi P, Eisele J, Ettinger LJ, DiMichele D. Nephrotic Syndrome as a Complication of Immune Tolerance in Hemophilia B. Blood. 1997;89(3):1115–5.

Part II
Rare Factor Deficiencies

Manifestations and Treatment of Congenital Fibrinogen Deficiency

Ruchika Sharma and Bryce A. Kerlin

Case Presentation A pediatric intern was called from the nursery about a newborn baby boy with continued bleeding from the umbilical cord. The neonate was born full term, via spontaneous vaginal delivery without instrumentation or other complications. The baby's Apgar scores were 8 and 9 at 1 and 5 minutes, respectively. The mother is 26 years old, gravida 1, now para 1, without known health problems. On physical exam, the neonate has an umbilical cord hematoma with some oozing. His vital signs are normal for age.

R. Sharma
Medical College of Wisconsin, Versiti Wisconsin, Milwaukee, WI, USA
e-mail: rsharma@versiti.org

B. A. Kerlin (✉)
Nationwide Children's Hospital, Division of Pediatric Hematology, Oncology and Bone Marrow Transplant, Columbus, OH, USA

Department of Pediatrics, The Ohio State University College of Medicine, Columbus, OH, USA

Center for Clinical and Translational Research, Abigail Wexner Research Institute, Columbus, OH, USA
e-mail: bryce.kerlin@nationwidechildrens.org

© Springer Nature Switzerland AG 2020
A. L. Dunn et al. (eds.), *Pediatric Bleeding Disorders*,
https://doi.org/10.1007/978-3-030-31661-7_5

Multiple Choice Management Question

You suspect he may have a bleeding disorder. The next step you perform is:

1. **Obtain CBC, PT/PTT, and fibrinogen**.
2. Administer FFP to stop the bleeding.
3. Apply pressure on the umbilical cord.
4. Give a blood transfusion.

Differential Diagnosis

The differential diagnoses for this male neonate include hemophilia A and B, thrombocytopenia, rare factor deficiencies, fibrinogen problems, von Willebrand disease, and platelet dysfunction.

Laboratory Findings

A CBC was performed demonstrating a normal white count, differential, and platelet count. His hemoglobin was 10.5 g/dl. His PT was 18.2 seconds and PTT was 45 seconds which were both prolonged for age. The fibrinogen level was 15 mg/dL. A thrombin time was performed to further evaluate the fibrinogen and was prolonged at 24 seconds.

Clinical Manifestations of Fibrinogen Disorders

Fibrinogen is a complex glycoprotein that polymerizes following cleavage by thrombin to form the fibrin clot. It is also the primary ligand for the platelet integrin $\alpha_{IIb}\beta_3$ which mediates aggregation of activated platelets. Congenital fibrinogen disorders are heterogeneous and comprise two classes of fibrinogen defects: type I, afibrinogenemia or hypofibrinogenemia, in which there are absent or low plasma fibrinogen antigen levels (quantitative fibrinogen deficiencies), and type II, dysfibrinogenemia or hypo-dysfibrinogenemia, in which there are normal or reduced antigen levels associated with disproportionately low functional activity (qualitative fibrinogen deficiencies) [1]. In 1920, two German physicians described the first case of congenital afibrinogenemia in a 9-year-old boy experiencing bleeding episodes from early childhood [2]. The common manifestations of afibrinogenemia are umbilical stump bleeding (which can be life-threatening) and bleeding from mucosal surfaces, particularly heavy menstrual bleeding, epistaxis, and bleeding in the oral cavity [3]. Other manifestations include musculoskeletal bleeding (including hemarthroses) and bleeding with minor surgeries or trauma. Bleeding in most cases of congenital dysfibrinogenemia is generally milder than afibrinogenemia [4]. Because fibrinogen is necessary for both hemostasis and thrombosis, defects in this protein may be associated with a bleeding phenotype, thrombotic phenotype, or both [3–5]. Women with fibrinogen defects may suffer from heavy menstrual bleeding, excessive postpartum bleeding, spontaneous pregnancy loss, or thrombotic complications. Table 5.1 summarizes the clinical manifestations of these fibrinogen disorders.

Laboratory Diagnosis

In many cases, the diagnosis is suspected by the combination of both a prolonged prothrombin time (PT) and activated partial thromboplastin time (aPTT). Fibrinogen levels are most often assessed using the clotting-based Clauss method (sometimes referred to as the "clottable" fibrinogen level). Alternatively, an immunological method (such as an enzyme-linked immunosorbent assay) may be utilized. A discrepancy between the clottable and immunologic fibrinogen levels or a ratio of functional activity to antigen lower than 0.7 is suggestive of dysfibrinogenemia [6]. In quantitative fibrinogen deficiencies, such as afibrinogenemia or hypofibrinogenemia, both the clottable and immunologic levels will be concordantly absent or decreased, respectively. The thrombin

Table 5.1 Comparison chart of subtypes of congenital fibrinogen disorders

	Afibrinogenemia	Hypofibrinogenemia	Dysfibrinogenemia
Transmission	Autosomal recessive	Autosomal dominant or recessive	Autosomal dominant or recessive
Impact	5 in 10 million	Less than afibrinogenemia	1 in 1 million
Plasma fibrinogen level	<20 mg/dl	20–80 mg/dl	200–400 mg/dl
Symptoms	Umbilical cord bleeding Mucocutaneous bleeding Gastrointestinal hemorrhage Intracranial bleeding Articular bleeding (in 20% of subjects)	Umbilical cord bleeding Mucocutaneous bleeding Gastrointestinal hemorrhage Intracranial bleeding (infrequent) Articular bleeding (in 20% of subjects)	Bleeding, thrombosis, or both
Treatment	Fibrinogen	Fibrinogen	Fibrinogen or Anticoagulant

Adapted from the Canadian Hemophilia Society. Website link: http://www.hemophilia.ca/en/bleeding-disorders/other-factor-deficiencies/factor-i-deficiency%2D%2Dfibrinogen-deficiency time will be prolonged in both quantitative and qualitative defects. Of note, the thrombin time is highly sensitive to heparin contamination, and a reptilase time (not prolonged with heparin) may be utilized in this setting to exclude a specimen quality issue. Thromboelastography has also been described to characterize variable deficiencies of fibrinogen but is not clinically utilized [7].

Epidemiology and Inheritance

Congenital fibrinogen disorders result from mutations in any of the three genes (*FGA*, *FGB*, and *FGG*) that encode the three polypeptide chains of fibrinogen (Aα, Bβ, and γ; as shown in Fig. 5.1) and are located in a 50 kb region on chromosome 4q31.3 [9]. Afibrinogenemia is a rare autosomal recessive disorder, with an estimated prevalence of 1 or 2 per 1,000,000. Both homozygous and compound heterozygous forms are described. Congenital dysfibrinogenemia is generally associated with autosomal dominant inheritance caused by heterozygosity for missense mutations, while other mutations have also been reported [9]. Some mutations may predict phenotype, and some variants are associated with thrombotic risk.

Management Options

Replacement therapy is the mainstay of treatment for bleeding episodes and includes plasma-derived fibrinogen concentrate, cryoprecipitate, and fresh frozen plasma (FFP). Long-term secondary prophylaxis has been described after CNS hemorrhage. Plasma-derived human fibrinogen concentrate is approved for the treatment of congenital fibrinogen deficiency, and the efficacy and safety of a new human fibrinogen concentrate is also being studied [10, 11]. In centers where fibrinogen concentrates are unavailable, cryoprecipitate is a reasonable alternative as it contains higher concentration of fibrinogen than FFP. For mild mucocutaneous bleeding symptoms or minor surgical procedures, agents such as antifibrinolytics may also be utilized. Topical treatments such as

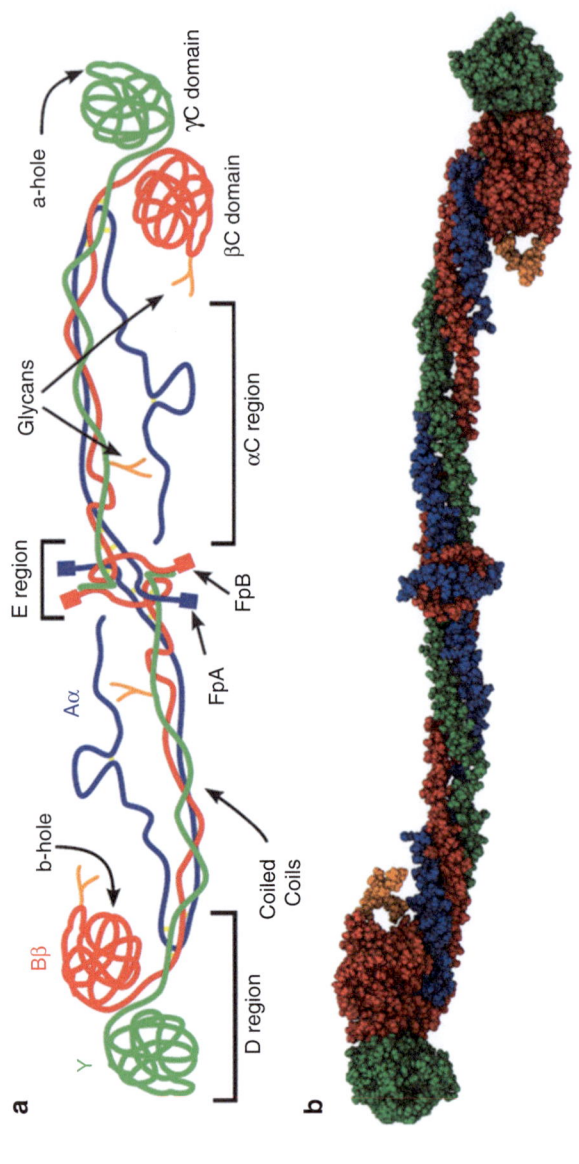

Fig. 5.1 Schematic representation of the fibrinogen molecule with Van der Waals representation of the crystallographic structure. (Köhler et al. [8]. "Reproduced with permission")

topical thrombin or fibrin glue may also be beneficial in the trauma or surgical settings. In women with congenital fibrinogen disorders, pregnancy must be managed with caution while providing replacement therapy and monitoring for reported thromboembolic complications; some women may also need concomitant anticoagulant therapy [12]. For patients with dysfibrinogenemias and others with a thrombotic phenotype, a careful review of the personal and family history is recommended for making management decisions regarding anticoagulation.

Outcomes and Follow-Up

Patients with qualitative and quantitative defects of fibrinogen, particularly afibrinogenemias, may benefit from being seen in comprehensive multidisciplinary clinics at various federally funded hemophilia treatment centers (HTCs). Patients should be followed at least annually for improved outcomes.

Clinical Pearls and Pitfalls

- Clinical manifestations of congenital fibrinogen disorders are heterogeneous and may be associated with bleeding, thrombosis, or both.
- Both autosomal recessive and dominant forms exist.
- Evaluation includes assessment of both the fibrinogen antigen and the activity.
- Management includes prevention of bleeding events and use of antifibrinolytics, FFP, cryoprecipitate, and fibrinogen concentrates.
- Patients with severe bleeding phenotypes are best served by specialized hemophilia treatment centers.

References

1. de Moerloose P, Casini A, Neerman-Arbez M. Congenital fibrinogen disorders: an update. Semin Thromb Hemost. 2013;39:585–95.
2. Rabe F, Solomon E. Ueber Faserstoffmangel im Blute bei einen Falle von Hämophile. Arch Klin Med. 1920;132:240–4.
3. Lak M, Keihani M, Elahi F, Peyvandi F, Mannucci PM. Bleeding and thrombosis in 55 patients with inherited afibrinogenaemia. Br J Haematol. 1999;107(1):204–6.
4. Shapiro SE, Phillips E, Manning RA, Morse CV, Murden SL, Laffan MA, Mumford AD. Clinical phenotype, laboratory features and genotype of 35 patients with heritable dysfibrinogenaemia. Br J Haematol. 2013;160:220–7.
5. Hanss M, Biot F. A database for human fibrinogen variants. Ann N Y Acad Sci. 2001;936:89–90.
6. Krammer B, Anders O, Nagel HR, Burstein C, Steiner M. Screening of dysfibrinogenaemia using the fibrinogen function versus antigen concentration ratio. Thromb Res. 1994;76:577–9.
7. Galanakis DK, Neerman-Arbez M, Brennan S, et al. Thromboelastographic phenotypes of fibrinogen and its variants: clinical and non-clinical implications. Thromb Res. 2014 Jun;133(6):1115–23.
8. Köhler S, Schmid F, Settanni G. The internal dynamics of fibrinogen and its implications for coagulation and adsorption. PLoS Comput Biol. 2015;11(9):e1004346.
9. Tiscia GL, Margaglione M. Human fibrinogen: molecular and genetic aspects of congenital disorders. Int J Mol Sci. 2018;19:1597.
10. Kreuz W, Meili E, Peter-Salonen K, et al. Efficacy and tolerability of a pasteurized human fibrinogen concentrate in patients with congenital fibrinogen deficiency. Transfus Apher Sci. 2005;32:247–53.
11. Lissitchkov T, Madan B, Djambas Khayat C, et al. Efficacy and safety of a new human fibrinogen concentrate in patients with congenital fibrinogen deficiency: an interim analysis of a phase III trial. Transfusion. 2018 Feb;58(2):413–22.
12. Casini A, Neerman-Arbez M, Ariëns RA, de Moerloose P. Dysfibrinogenemia: from molecular anomalies to clinical manifestations and management. J Thromb Haemost. 2015 Jun;13(6):909–19.

Diagnosis and Management of FVII Deficiency

6

Ruchika Sharma and Bryce A. Kerlin

Case Presentation A 15-year-old female presents to your clinic with heavy menstrual bleeding. On further questioning, she also endorses a history of easy bruising and recurrent epistaxis. There is a family history of heavy menstrual bleeding in her mother and maternal grandmother. On physical examination, she is a normal-sized female with extensive bruising on her lower extremities. She has mild conjunctival pallor. Her vital signs are normal for age.

R. Sharma
Medical College of Wisconsin, Versiti Wisconsin, Milwaukee, WI, USA
e-mail: rsharma@versiti.org

B. A. Kerlin (✉)
Nationwide Children's Hospital, Division of Pediatric Hematology, Oncology and Bone Marrow Transplant, Columbus, OH, USA

Department of Pediatrics, The Ohio State University College of Medicine, Columbus, OH, USA

Center for Clinical and Translational Research, Abigail Wexner Research Institute, Columbus, OH, USA
e-mail: bryce.kerlin@nationwidechildrens.org

© Springer Nature Switzerland AG 2020
A. L. Dunn et al. (eds.), *Pediatric Bleeding Disorders*,
https://doi.org/10.1007/978-3-030-31661-7_6

Multiple-Choice Management Question

You suspect that she may have a bleeding disorder. Do you:

1. Refer her to gynecology
2. **Perform a CBC, PT, and PTT**
3. Refer to hematology

Differential Diagnoses

The differential diagnoses for this girl include thrombocytopenia, factor deficiencies, symptomatic hemophilia carrier state, hypo/dysfibrinogenemia, von Willebrand disease, and platelet dysfunction.

Laboratory Findings

A CBC was performed that showed normal white count, differential, and platelet count. Her hemoglobin was mildly decreased at 10.5 g/dl. Her PT was 18.1 seconds and PTT 35 seconds. A PT mixing study was performed which corrected to 13 seconds. Evaluation for levels of coagulation factors of the extrinsic clotting pathway was performed including factors II, V, VII, and X coagulant activity levels. All others were normal except a FVII activity level of 14 IU/dl.

Diagnosis and Assessment

Factor VII (FVII) is a plasma vitamin K-dependent serine protease produced by the liver [1]. The activated form of FVII (FVIIa) interacts with tissue factor (TF) exposed on the vascular lumen upon injury and initiates blood coagulation as shown in Fig. 6.1 [2]. The FVIIa–TF complex further activates factors IX (to FIXa) and X (to FXa), which induce the downstream formation of a stable fibrin clot.

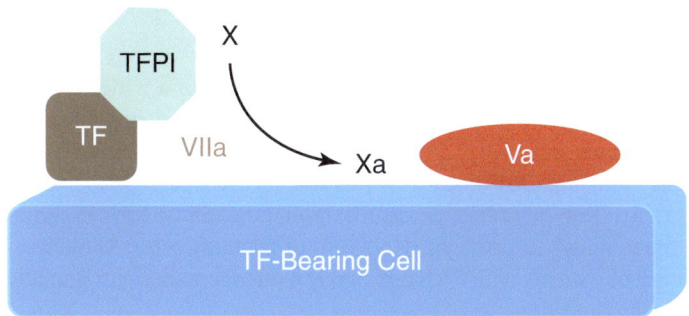

Fig. 6.1 Activated factor VII (FVIIa)–tissue factor (TF) complex causes propagation of coagulation

Diagnosis of factor VII deficiency may be made during evaluation for bleeding symptoms, screening of members of a family with history of factor VII deficiency, or during workup for an isolated prolonged prothrombin time (PT). An isolated prolonged PT, which further corrects on mixing studies, is suspicious for deficiency of vitamin K-dependent factors. A factor VII activity assay is used for diagnosing FVII deficiency. FVII coagulant activity is determined with a one-stage PT assay mixing citrated patient plasma sample, FVII-deficient reagent plasma, and thromboplastin.

Genetic Diagnosis

The FVII gene (*F7*) is located on chromosome 13q34, and mutations of the *F7* gene have been characterized in the vast majority of FVII-deficient patients [3]. Most FVII mutations are missense mutations, and most are in the catalytic domain. There is evidence for phenotypic heterogeneity even in the presence of identical FVII gene mutations [4]. Although not routinely performed, there may be a role for carrier testing by gene sequencing, in patients with a questionable diagnosis and for prenatal diagnosis (cord blood) in families with a history of severe or life-threatening bleeding episodes.

Clinical Manifestations

Most patients with FVII deficiency present with a wide range of bleeding symptoms, most commonly mucocutaneous bleeding symptoms including epistaxis (60%), gingival bleeding (34%), easy bruising (36%), and heavy menstrual bleeding (69% females) [1, 5]. Ten to fifteen percent exhibit potentially life- or limb-threatening hemorrhages (CNS, GI, or hemarthrosis). About one-third of patients with FVII deficiency tend to remain asymptomatic during their life.

There is a lack of correlation between clinical phenotypes and FVII coagulant activity. Generally, FVII activity levels above 20% are considered to protect from spontaneous bleeding [6]. However, even in asymptomatic individuals, certain situations such as major surgery may cause excessive bleeding and may warrant prophylactic or therapeutic measures [7].

Epidemiology, Inheritance

Inherited factor VII deficiency is the most common of the rare, autosomal recessive bleeding disorders with an estimated prevalence of 1 in 500,000. FVII deficiency may be divided into two categories: type I defects (quantitative, with decreased FVII coagulant activity and FVII antigen, FVII:Ag) generally result from nonsense or deletions of all or a portion of the gene; meanwhile, type II (qualitative, with low FVII activity and normal FVII:Ag) defects generally arise from missense mutations which alter the enzymatic function of the protein.

Acquired FVII deficiency may be seen in vitamin K deficiency, liver disease, or secondary to vitamin K antagonistic medications such as warfarin. Rarely, acquired coagulation inhibitors may be observed causing increased peripheral clearance of FVII seen in infections, autoimmune disorders, malignancy, and hematological stem cell transplantation [8].

Management Options

Therapeutic options for treatment of FVII deficiency may include recombinant coagulation factor VIIa (FVIIa), fresh frozen plasma (FFP), prothrombin complex concentrates (PCC), and antifibrinolytic therapies. Factor VII concentrates are most utilized for severe spontaneous bleeding episodes, major surgery, and prophylaxis. FFP is more readily available but may have side effects of causing volume overload and allergic reactions. For mild bleeding in patients with non-severe deficiency or as an adjunct to other therapies in severe patients, antifibrinolytic agents, such as aminocaproic acid and tranexamic acid, may also be utilized to stabilize the fibrin clot. Multicenter observational studies such as the Seven Treatment Evaluations Registry (STER) have provided evidence regarding indications, efficacy, and safety as well as schedules for replacement therapy for spontaneous bleeding episodes, major surgery, invasive procedures, and prophylaxis [9].

Outcomes and Follow-Up

A network of federally funded comprehensive hemophilia treatment centers (HTCs) exists to enhance access to care for persons with hemophilia and other severe bleeding disorders. Patients with factor VII deficiency, particularly severe FVII deficiency, may benefit by referral to one of these comprehensive multidisciplinary clinics with specialists in the care of patients with bleeding disorders. Patients should be followed at least annually in an HTC for optimal outcomes.

> **Clinical Pearls and Pitfalls**
> - Factor VII deficiency may manifest while evaluating an isolated prolonged PT.
> - Most patients with FVII deficiency present with mucocutaneous bleeding symptoms.

- Congenital FVII deficiency is a rare autosomal recessive disorder, and acquired forms are also seen.
- Treatment options include recombinant FVIIa, FFP, PCC, and antifibrinolytic agents.
- Patients are best managed in an HTC.

References

1. Mariani G, Bernardi F. Factor VII deficiency. Semin Thromb Hemost. 2009;35:400–6.
2. Butenas S, van't Veer C, Mann KG. "Normal" thrombin generation. Blood. 1999;94:2169–78.
3. McVey JH, Boswell E, Mumford AD, Kemball-Cook G, Tuddenham EG. Factor VII deficiency and the FVII mutation database. Hum Mutat. 2001;17:3–17.
4. Castoldi E, Govers-Riemslag JW, Pinotti M, et al. Coinheritance of factor V (FV) Leiden enhances thrombin formation and is associated with a mild bleeding phenotype in patients homozygous for the FVII 9726þ5G>A (FVII Lazio) mutation. Blood. 2003;102:4014–20.
5. Mariani G, Herrmann FH, Dolce A, Batorova A, Etro D, Peyvandi F, Wulff K, Schved JF, Auerswald G, Ingerslev J, et al. Clinical phenotypes and factor VII genotype in congenital factor VII deficiency. Thromb Haemost. 2005;93:481–7.
6. Perry DJ. Factor VII deficiency. Br J Haematol. 2002;118:689–700.
7. Benlakhal F, Mura T, Schved JF, Giansily-Blaizot M. A retrospective analysis of 157 surgical procedures performed without replacement therapy in 83 unrelated factor VII-deficient patients. J Thromb Haemost. 2011;9:1149–56.
8. Mulliez SM, Devreese KM. Isolated acquired factor VII deficiency: review of the literature. Acta Clin Belg. 2016 Apr;71(2):63–70.
9. Napolitano M, Giansily-Blaizot M, Dolce A, et al. Prophylaxis in congenital factor VII deficiency: indications, efficacy and safety. Results from the Seven Treatment Evaluation Registry (STER). Haematologica. 2013;98(4):538–44.

Approach to Mucosal Bleeding in an Adolescent with FXI Deficiency

Ruchika Sharma and Bryce A. Kerlin

Case Presentation A 13-year-old male was referred from the dental clinic for prolonged bleeding after wisdom tooth extraction. He endorses no prior history of unexplained bleeding. On further questioning, he is of Ashkenazi Jewish descent. There is a family history of heavy menstrual bleeding in his mother, and she also has a history of excessive bleeding after a tonsillectomy surgery. On physical examination, he is a normal-sized male with continued oozing from his site of tooth extraction. His vital signs are normal for age.

R. Sharma
Medical College of Wisconsin, Versiti Wisconsin, Milwaukee, WI, USA
e-mail: rsharma@versiti.org

B. A. Kerlin (✉)
Nationwide Children's Hospital, Division of Pediatric Hematology, Oncology and Bone Marrow Transplant, Columbus, OH, USA

Department of Pediatrics, The Ohio State University College of Medicine, Columbus, OH, USA

Center for Clinical and Translational Research, Abigail Wexner Research Institute, Columbus, OH, USA
e-mail: bryce.kerlin@nationwidechildrens.org

Multiple-Choice Management Question

You suspect he may have a bleeding disorder. The next step you perform is:

1. Obtain CBC, PT/PTT.
2. **Administer FFP to stop the bleeding**.
3. Administer aFVII to stop the bleeding.
4. Give a blood transfusion.

Differential Diagnoses

The differential diagnoses for this boy include hemophilia A and B, thrombocytopenia, other factor deficiencies, hypo/dysfibrinogenemia, von Willebrand disease, and platelet dysfunction.

Laboratory Findings

A CBC was performed that showed normal white count, differential, and platelet count. His hemoglobin was 12.5 g/dl. His PT was 14.1 seconds and PTT 56 seconds. A 1:1 PTT mixing study was performed which showed correction to 35 seconds. Evaluation for levels of coagulation factors of the intrinsic pathway were performed including factors VIII, IX, XI, and XII coagulant activity levels. All of which were normal except for FXI activity of 10 IU/dl.

Diagnosis and Assessment

Factor XI (FXI) is the zymogen of a serine protease enzyme in the intrinsic pathway of blood coagulation and is an important factor in the creation of a stable fibrin clot. FXI is activated by thrombin and further reinforces the intrinsic clotting pathway by activation of factor IX as shown in Fig. 7.1 [1, 2]. FXI is produced in the

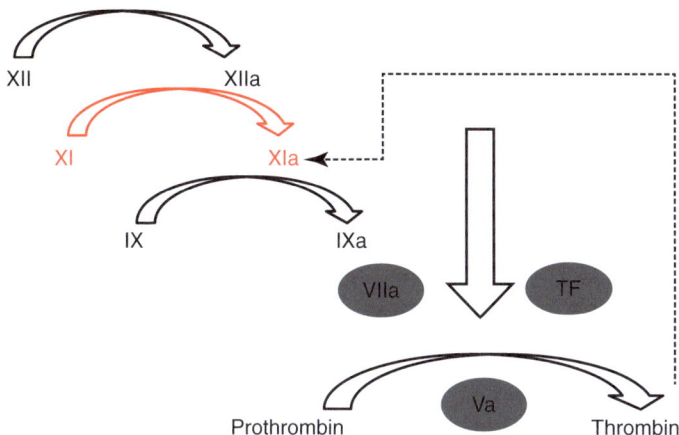

Fig. 7.1 Scheme for the cascade/waterfall model of thrombin generation triggered by activation of FXII. The dotted line indicates feedback activation of FXI by thrombin. (Adapted from Gailani et al. [2])

liver and circulates in the bloodstream as a homodimer complexed with high-molecular-weight kininogen.

Clinical Manifestations

Factor XI (FXI) deficiency is a rare, autosomal disorder (mostly autosomal recessive). Homozygous or compound heterozygous patients have severe deficiency ($\leq$15 IU/dL), whereas heterozygotes have partial deficiency (16–60 IU/dL) [3, 4]. This classification does not reflect bleeding risk since many individuals with very low FXI levels do not bleed. Patients with all levels of FXI deficiency can present with bleeding following surgery or injury; however, spontaneous bleeding is rare. Bleeding typically occurs at sites with high fibrinolytic activity (mouth, nose, genitourinary tract) and can also include heavy menstrual bleeding, intracerebral hemorrhage, and gastrointestinal bleeding [1–3]. FXI deficiency can also occur in patients with Noonan syndrome, which is a disorder characterized by a wide spectrum of symptoms and physical features.

Epidemiology, Inheritance

The estimated prevalence of severe FXI deficiency in most populations is ~1 in 1 million but is higher in Ashkenazi Jews where heterozygosity approaches 8% [1, 3]. Factor XI deficiency has also been reported in non-Jewish patients, including patients of Japanese, Korean, Chinese, German, Italian, African American, English, Indian, and Arab ancestry [3, 5]. Patients with similar FXI laboratory tests including FXI antigen, FXI/clotting (FXI:C) activity, or activated partial thromboplastin time (aPTT) exhibit variable bleeding tendencies, and these vary even within individuals of the same genotype [5–7]. Recently, plasma clot formation and fibrinolysis assays have been shown to predict bleeding tendency in an independent cohort of patients with severe and partial FXI deficiency [8].

Mutation Subtypes

The *FXI* gene was identified in 1987 and is located on chromosome 4 [9]. Three independent point mutations in the factor *XI* gene were identified to be responsible for the majority of cases of FXI deficiency in Ashkenazi Jews [3]. These mutations were designated Types I, II, and III. The Type I mutation is least prevalent. The Type II mutation is the nonsense mutation Glu117Stop, and the type III mutation is the missense mutation Phe283Leu. Homozygotes for the Glu117Stop mutation produce no FXI and have a higher bleeding risk than homozygotes for Phe283Leu whose baseline level approximates 10 IU/dL. In the past two decades, more than 220 mutations in the FXI gene have been reported in patients with FXI deficiency, of which 7 have shown a founder effect [6].

Management Options

Therapy for prevention of bleeding during surgery in patients with severe FXI deficiency consists of plasma, factor XI concentrates, fibrin glue, and antifibrinolytic agents [4].

Replacement therapy should be considered in high-risk situations, especially when FXI levels are below 20 IU/dL. Efficacy and safety of a FXI concentrate has been demonstrated in a phase 3 prospective French study, but is not available in the United States [10]. Inhibitors to FXI develop in one-third of patients with severe FXI deficiency, particularly in patients with null-allele mutations, following exposure to plasma, FXI concentrates, or anti-RhD immunoglobulin [6, 11]. In patients with an inhibitor to FXI, recombinant factor VIIa may be useful.

Outcomes and Follow-Up

Patients with factor XI deficiency, particularly severe XI deficiency, may benefit from being seen in comprehensive multidisciplinary clinics at various federally funded hemophilia treatment centers (HTCs). Patients should be followed at least annually in an HTC for improved outcomes.

> **Clinical Pearls and Pitfalls**
> - Factor XI deficiency is most prevalent among Ashkenazi Jews.
> - Spontaneous bleeding is rare, and many patients are asymptomatic or may exhibit bleeding at the sites of high fibrinolytic activity.
> - Bleeding tendencies are variable and do not correlate with factor XI activity levels.
> - Patients with severe FXI deficiency should be followed at least annually in an HTC for improved outcomes.

References

1. Shapiro AD, Peyvandi F. Rare coagulation disorders resource room. Available at: https://www.rarecoagulationdisorders.org/. Accessed October 10th, 2018.
2. Emsley J, McEwan PA, Gailani D. Structure and function of factor XI. Blood. 2010;115(13):2569–77.

3. Asakai R, Chung DW, Davie EW, Seligsohn U. Factor XI deficiency in Ashkenazi Jews in Israel. N Engl J Med. 1991;325(3):153–8.
4. Seligsohn U. Factor XI deficiency in humans. J Thromb Haemost. 2009;7(suppl):184–7.
5. Ragni MV, Sinha D, Seaman F, Lewis JH, Spero JA, Walsh PN. Comparison of bleeding tendency, factor XI coagulant activity, and factor XI antigen in 25 factor XI-deficient kindreds. Blood. 1985;65:719–24.
6. Duga S, Salomon O. Congenital factor XI deficiency: an update. Semin Thromb Hemost. 2013;39(6):621–31.
7. Peyvandi F, Palla R, Menegatti M, et al; European Network of Rare Bleeding Disorders Group. Coagulation factor activity and clinical bleeding severity in rare bleeding disorders: results from the European Network of Rare Bleeding Disorders. J Thromb Haemost. 2012;10(4):615–621.
8. Gidley GN, Holle LA, Burthem J, Bolton-Maggs PHB, Lin F-C, Wolberg AS. Abnormal plasma clot formation and fibrinolysis reveal bleeding tendency in patients with partial factor XI deficiency. Blood Adv. 2018;2:1076–88.
9. Asakai R, Davie EW, Chung DW. Organization of the gene for human factor XI. Biochemistry. 1987;26:7221–8.
10. Bauduer F, de Raucourt E, Boyer-Neumann C, et al. Factor XI replacement for inherited factor XI deficiency in routine clinical practice: results of the HEMOLEVEN prospective 3-year postmarketing study. Haemophilia. 2015 Jul;21(4):481–9.
11. Salomon O, Zivelin A, Livnat T, et al. Prevalence, causes, and characterization of factor XI inhibitors in patients with inherited factor XI deficiency. Blood. 2003;101(12):4783–8.

Recognition and Care of a Newborn with FXIII Deficiency

8

Bryce A. Kerlin

Case Presentation A 10-day-old female presents to the emergency department with pallor, tachycardia, and oozing hemorrhage from the umbilical navel. The infant's mother explains that the bleeding began when the umbilical stump detached 2 days ago. Her pediatrician advised that she bring the infant to the emergency room because the bleeding has not stopped despite multiple first aid attempts, including attempted silver nitrate cautery at the pediatrician's office. With each attempt, the bleeding has stopped, only to be observed again several hours later. This is the mother's third baby. Two older siblings, a 4-year-old boy and a 3-year-old girl, are both healthy. The mother denies any bleeding symptoms

---

B. A. Kerlin (✉)
Nationwide Children's Hospital, Division of Pediatric Hematology, Oncology and Bone Marrow Transplant, Columbus, OH, USA

Department of Pediatrics, The Ohio State University College of Medicine, Columbus, OH, USA

Center for Clinical and Translational Research, Abigail Wexner Research Institute, Columbus, OH, USA
e-mail: bryce.kerlin@nationwidechildrens.org

© Springer Nature Switzerland AG 2020
A. L. Dunn et al. (eds.), *Pediatric Bleeding Disorders*,
https://doi.org/10.1007/978-3-030-31661-7_8

for either of her other children. She has had no personal bleeding symptoms, including easy bruising, epistaxis, gum bleeding, and heavy menses, and no surgical bleeding problems. Similarly, she denies that the infant's father or other members of an extended family history have bleeding difficulties. The mother affirms that the baby did receive a dose of vitamin K before discharge from the delivery hospital. You arrange for a packed red blood cell transfusion and admission to the hematology service for further management.

Multiple-Choice Management Question

You suspect that the baby may have a bleeding disorder, as a next step you:

A. Order a prothrombin time (PT), activated partial thromboplastin time (aPTT), and fibrinogen
B. Order a factor XIII activity assay
C. Arrange for transfusion of cryoprecipitate 5 mL/kg
D. Arrange for transfusion of fresh frozen plasma (FFP) 10 mL/kg
E. A and C
F. B and D
G. **A, B, and C**
H. A, B, and D

Differential Diagnosis

The differential diagnosis for an infant presenting with bleeding from the umbilical stump includes nonhemorrhagic disorders, such as cellulitis, but the most common etiologies are congenital coagulation defects. If the child was a boy, hemophilia (A or B) might be considered, but umbilical bleeding is only observed in about 2% of infants with hemophilia [1]. Umbilical hemorrhage is a relatively common presentation for fibrinogen mutations but is essentially pathognomonic for congenital factor XIII (FXIII) deficiency. Umbilical hemorrhage is rarely reported among the other rare coagulation factor deficiencies.

Laboratory Findings

Patients with factor FXIII deficiency are expected to have normal blood counts in the absence of chronic blood loss, which may lead to anemia. The prothrombin time (PT), activated partial thromboplastin time (aPTT), thrombin time, and fibrinogen are generally normal unless an acute major hemorrhage (e.g., intracranial hemorrhage) has initiated an episode of disseminated intravascular coagulopathy (DIC) with associated consumptive coagulopathy. Thus, specific factor XIII assays must be pursued to make an accurate and timely diagnosis [2]. Qualitative assays of factor XIII activity, using clot solubility assays (e.g., the 5 M urea lysis assay) are widely available but have limited sensitivity and are thus no longer recommended [3]. Therefore, while these assays may provide a relatively quick, locally available diagnosis, a negative result should not be relied upon to exclude the diagnosis. It is thus highly recommended that a kinetic enzyme assay be utilized to accurately determine the factor XIII activity of the patient's plasma. The International Society on Thrombosis and Haemostasis (ISTH) has recommended a testing algorithm for definitive diagnosis (Fig. 8.1) [2, 3].

Epidemiology and Inheritance

Factor XIII circulates as a heterotetramer consisting of two FXIII A-subunits and two FXIII B-subunits (Fig. 8.2). The B-subunits act as carriers which prolong the half-life of the A-subunit proenzyme. A-subunits are activated upon thrombin-mediated proteolytic cleavage which removes the activation peptide and, in the presence of calcium, dissociates the B-subunits to generate the fully activated FXIII A_2 homodimer (FXIII-A_2*; Fig. 8.2).

Activated factor XIII (FXIII-A_2*) is the only known transglutaminase enzyme of the coagulation system. Whereas most of the coagulation enzymes are serine proteases (e.g., the vitamin K-dependent factors) or catalysts that bring the proteases into proximity with their substrates (e.g., factors V and VIII),

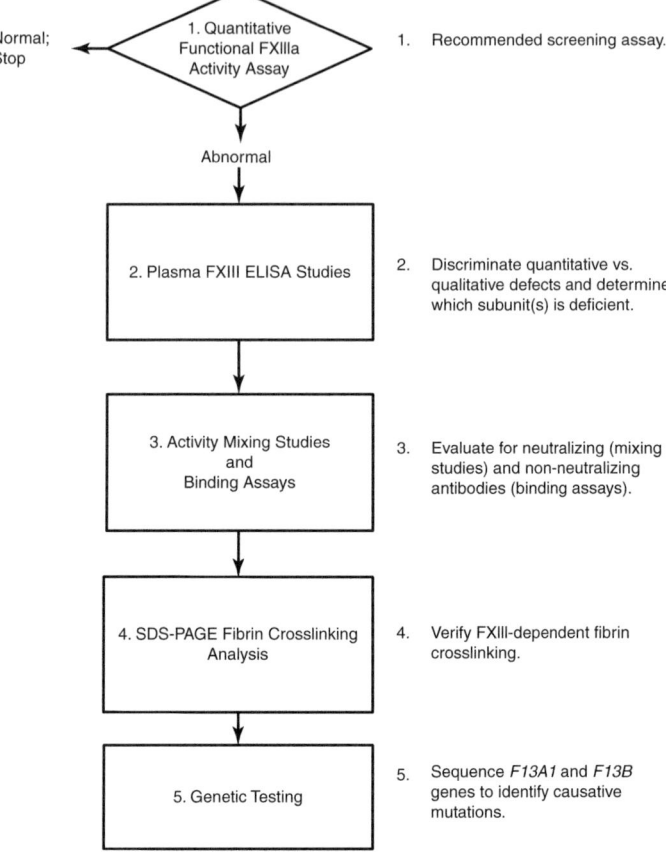

Fig. 8.1 Diagnostic algorithm for suspected factor XIII deficiency as proposed by the International Society on Thrombosis and Haemostasis (ISTH) [3]

factor XIII links its protein substrates together via the formation of ε-N-(γ-glutamyl)-lysyl covalent bonds which results in an isopeptide bond between a glutamine residue of one substrate and an amino terminus or amino sidechain of the second substrate. Its primary physiologic function is to stabilize the fibrin clot by crosslinking fibrin γ- and α-chains to form γ_2-dimers, high-molecular-weight α_2-dimers, and α-γ polymers. Perhaps most importantly,

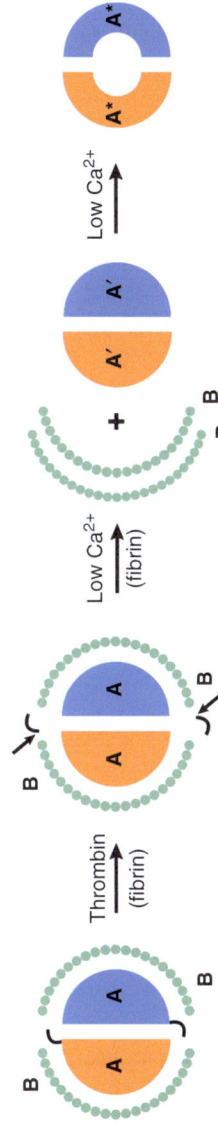

Fig. 8.2 Schematic representation of factor XIII activation biochemistry

FXIII-A$_2$* catalyzes cross-links between fibrin α-chains and α2-antiplasmin, thereby directly incorporating a potent fibrinolysis inhibitor directly into the forming fibrin clot and thus enhancing its resistance to premature fibrinolysis [4].

Severe, congenital FXIII deficiency is an autosomal recessive rare bleeding disorder that affects ~1 in 2 million people [5]. The prevalence may be higher in the setting of consanguineous reproduction and is particularly high in the Sistan and Baluchestan Province of southeastern Iran due to a founder mutation in the region [6]. Factor XIII deficiency can be caused by deficiency of either FXIII-A or FXIII-B. B-subunit deficiency results in dramatic shortening of the FXIII-A circulating half-life due to reduced protection from spontaneous FXIII-A proteolysis (similar to the mechanism by which von Willebrand factor protects circulating factor VIII). Factor XIII-B deficiency is the least common form of the disease, having been described in fewer than 20 kindreds [7, 8]. Thus, FXIII-A deficiency is the most commonly observed form of the disease. In addition to congenital deficiency, autoimmune and consumptive forms of FXIII deficiency have also been described [2].

Management Options

The vast majority of children with congenital FXIII deficiency (~80%) present with umbilical stump bleeding early in life, as in the above example [8]. Other common manifestations include bruising, hematomas, oral mucosa hemorrhage, menorrhagia, impaired wound healing, and recurrent spontaneous miscarriage. Perhaps most concerning, however, is the estimated 30% incidence of spontaneous, life-threatening intracranial hemorrhage. The latter manifestation is the major concern underlying primary prophylactic FXIII supplementation as the standard of care [9–16].

In comparison to fresh frozen plasma, factor XIII is enriched two- to three-fold in cryoprecipitate [17], containing an estimated 288 IU FXIII activity per bag (20–25 mL/bag). Because FXIII concentrates are often only stocked in tertiary care hospitals and hemophilia treatment centers, cryoprecipitate is often the most readily available first-line treatment product. Factor XIII recovery is ~2 IU/dL for every IU/kg administered; thus, a cryoprecipitate dose of 5 mL/kg will raise the FXIII activity of a severely deficient patient (0 IU/dL baseline activity) to 120–144 IU/dL (the upper quartile of the reference range). Of course, the use of cryoprecipitate is associated with the usual risks associated with blood product transfusions. Thus, once the diagnosis has been confirmed and adequate pharmacologic options secured, treatment should be transitioned to a purified FXIII concentrate product to limit these risks [11–14]. Plasma-derived FXIII concentrate (i.e. Corifact®; formerly "Fibrogammin P") consists of the FXIII-A_2B_2 heterodimer and is thus the only purified FXIII product available for the treatment of FXIII B-subunit deficiency. This product will also suffice for patients with A-subunit deficiency, who also have the option for treatment with recombinant FXIII-A_2 (i.e. Tretten® (USA and Canada); NovoThirteen® (elsewhere)).

Antifibrinolytic therapy has limited utility in the setting of factor XIII deficiency due to the instability of the fibrin clot in the absence of FXIII-dependent crosslinking.

Outcomes and Follow-Up

Primary prophylaxis with a purified FXIII product should commence as early, after the diagnosis, as possible to prevent the potential for bleeding-related morbidity and mortality. Infused FXIII has an estimated half-life of ~10–14 days [5], enabling once-monthly dosing. Due to issues with the sensitivity of the commonly used assays and the lack of a World Health Organization (WHO) international FXIII standard before 2004 (enabling comparisons between published prophylaxis protocols), the optimal trough FXIII activity level remains controversial [5]. The recommended regimen for plasma-derived FXIII is 40 IU/kg every 28 days, adjusted to maintain a trough of 5–20 IU/dL. Meanwhile, the recommended regimen for recombinant FXIII-A_2 is 35 IU/kg every 28 days, targeting a trough of ≥ 10 IU/dL.

Patients receiving adequate prophylaxis have a very low incidence of nontraumatic, spontaneous bleeding [11–14]. Stable, uncomplicated patients on prophylaxis should be monitored once or twice yearly by a knowledgeable hematologist (e.g. at a federally funded hemophilia treatment center) to evaluate for evidence of occult bleeding and appropriate dose adjustments. Interval phone contact may be important to encourage adherence to the prophylactic regimen. Because bleeding events, surgery, and trauma may be associated with accelerated consumption of FXIII, additional doses may be required. Thus, it is prudent to obtain steady-state FXIII activity levels to determine individual pharmacokinetics. In the setting of surgery or trauma, levels should be obtained frequently to guide dose adjustments needed to provide adequate hemostasis.

Non-neutralizing anti-FXIII antibodies have been reported in patients on prophylaxis, but have not been associated with increased bleeding symptoms or treatment failure [18]. Inhibitors to FXIII are rare in congenital FXIII deficiency. However, acquired, autoimmune FXIII deficiency has been reported, particularly among the elderly [19]. Therefore, the possibility of clinically important FXIII antibodies cannot be completely negated.

Clinical Pearls and Pitfalls
- Factor XIII should be high on the differential for an infant with umbilical stump bleeding.
- The accurate and timely diagnosis of FXIII deficiency may enable lifesaving intervention with FXIII infusions.
- Though clot solubility tests are widely available, they must not be over-relied upon due to their lack of sensitivity and specificity.
- Because definitive testing is often sent to a reference lab, the results may not be available for several days. However, timely empiric treatment with a FXIII product should not be delayed while awaiting these test results, particularly in pathognomonic situations (e.g., umbilical bleeding) or in the setting of life-threatening bleeds (e.g., intracranial hemorrhage).

References

1. Kulkarni R, Presley RJ, Lusher JM, Shapiro AD, Gill JC, Manco-Johnson M, et al. Complications of haemophilia in babies (first two years of life): a report from the Centers for Disease Control and Prevention Universal Data Collection System. Haemophilia. 2017;23(2):207–14.
2. Durda MA, Wolberg AS, Kerlin BA. State of the art in factor XIII laboratory assessment. Transfus Apher Sci. 2018;57(6):700–4.
3. Kohler HP, Ichinose A, Seitz R, Ariens RA, Muszbek L, Factor X, et al. Diagnosis and classification of factor XIII deficiencies. J Thromb Haemost. 2011;9(7):1404–6.
4. Fraser SR, Booth NA, Mutch NJ. The antifibrinolytic function of factor XIII is exclusively expressed through alpha(2)-antiplasmin cross-linking. Blood. 2011;117(23):6371–4.
5. Kerlin B, Brand B, Inbal A, Halimeh S, Nugent D, Lundblad M, et al. Pharmacokinetics of recombinant factor XIII at steady state in patients with congenital factor XIII A-subunit deficiency. J Thromb Haemost. 2014;12(12):2038–43.
6. Dorgalaleh A, Naderi M, Hosseini MS, Alizadeh S, Hosseini S, Tabibian S, et al. Factor XIII deficiency in Iran: a comprehensive review of the literature. Semin Thromb Hemost. 2015;41(3):323–9.
7. World Federation of Hemophilia Report on the Annual Global Survey 2012. Montreal; 2013 December 2012.
8. Karimi M, Bereczky Z, Cohan N, Muszbek L. Factor XIII deficiency. Semin Thromb Hemost. 2009;35(4):426–38.
9. Bolton-Maggs PH, Perry DJ, Chalmers EA, Parapia LA, Wilde JT, Williams MD, et al. The rare coagulation disorders--review with guidelines for management from the United Kingdom Haemophilia Centre Doctors' Organisation. Haemophilia. 2004;10(5):593–628.
10. Brackmann HH, Egbring R, Ferster A, Fondu P, Girardel JM, Kreuz W, et al. Pharmacokinetics and tolerability of factor XIII concentrates prepared from human placenta or plasma: a crossover randomised study. Thromb Haemost. 1995;74(2):622–5.
11. Dreyfus M, Barrois D, Borg JY, Claeyssens S, Torchet MF, Arnuti B, et al. Successful long-term replacement therapy with FXIII concentrate (Fibrogammin((R)) P) for severe congenital factor XIII deficiency: a prospective multicentre study. J Thromb Haemost. 2011;9(6):1264–6.
12. Lusher J, Pipe SW, Alexander S, Nugent D. Prophylactic therapy with Fibrogammin P is associated with a decreased incidence of bleeding episodes: a retrospective study. Haemophilia. 2010;16(2):316–21.
13. Kerlin BA, Inbal A, Will A, Williams M, Garly ML, Jacobsen L, et al. Recombinant factor XIII prophylaxis is safe and effective in young children with congenital factor XIII-A deficiency: international phase 3b trial results. J Thromb Haemost. 2017;15(8):1601–6.

14. Carcao M, Altisent C, Castaman G, Fukutake K, Kerlin BA, Kessler C, et al. Recombinant FXIII (rFXIII-A2) prophylaxis prevents bleeding and allows for surgery in patients with congenital FXIII A-subunit deficiency. Thromb Haemost. 2018;118(3):451–60.
15. Nugent DJ. Prophylaxis in rare coagulation disorders – factor XIII deficiency. Thromb Res. 2006;118(Suppl 1):S23–8.
16. Mumford AD, Ackroyd S, Alikhan R, Bowles L, Chowdary P, Grainger J, et al. Guideline for the diagnosis and management of the rare coagulation disorders: a United Kingdom Haemophilia Centre Doctors' Organization guideline on behalf of the British Committee for Standards in Haematology. Br J Haematol. 2014;167(3):304–26.
17. Caudill JS, Nichols WL, Plumhoff EA, Schulte SL, Winters JL, Gastineau DA, et al. Comparison of coagulation factor XIII content and concentration in cryoprecipitate and fresh-frozen plasma. Transfusion. 2009;49(4):765–70.
18. Inbal A, Oldenburg J, Carcao M, Rosholm A, Tehranchi R, Nugent D. Recombinant factor XIII: a safe and novel treatment for congenital factor XIII deficiency. Blood. 2012;119(22):5111–7.
19. Ichinose A, Japanese Collaborative Research Group on AH. Autoimmune acquired factor XIII deficiency due to anti-factor XIII/13 antibodies: a summary of 93 patients. Blood Rev. 2017;31(1):37–45.

Part III

von Willebrand Disease

Classification and Management of Type 1 von Willebrand Disease

9

Dominder Kaur and Sarah H. O'Brien

Case Presentation You are seeing a 6-year-old girl in clinic today, referred to hematology for history of easy bruising and a workup initiated prior to tonsillectomy and adenoidectomy. She has a normal prothrombin time, mildly prolonged partial thromboplastin time at 36 seconds (per the lab reference), a ristocetin cofactor level of 25%, and a von Willebrand antigen level of 27%. Her factor VIII level is within the normal range (>50%) and so are

---

D. Kaur (✉)
Department of Pediatrics, Division of Pediatric Hematology/Oncology/Stem Cell Transplant, Columbia University Irving Medical Center, Children's Hospital of New York/New York Presbyterian Morgan Stanley Children's Hospital, New York, NY, USA
e-mail: dk3076@cumc.columbia.edu

S. H. O'Brien
Nationwide Children's Hospital, Division of Pediatric Hematology, Oncology and Bone Marrow Transplant, Columbus, OH, USA

Center for Innovation in Pediatric Practice, Abigail Wexner Research Institute at Nationwide Children's Hospital, Columbus, OH, USA

Department of Pediatrics, The Ohio State University College of Medicine, Columbus, OH, USA
e-mail: Sarah.Obrien@nationwidechildrens.org

© Springer Nature Switzerland AG 2020
A. L. Dunn et al. (eds.), *Pediatric Bleeding Disorders*,
https://doi.org/10.1007/978-3-030-31661-7_9

her multimers. All other bleeding workup was also normal, including her platelet count.

Multiple-Choice Management Question

The next steps in planning for her upcoming surgery include:

(a) Repeat von Willebrand profile to confirm diagnosis
(b) Set up a trial for assessing response to DDAVP
(c) **Both A and B**
(d) Neither of A and B and plan for surgery with Humate-P™ considering the invasiveness of the surgery

> Being a pre-surgical evaluation, we have enough time to complete the workup. This patient's labs are consistent with a type 1 VWD, with moderate levels. Next steps will be to confirm the diagnosis and set up a desmopressin/DDAVP trial as DDAVP can be a viable therapeutic option (option c). The upcoming procedure should be postponed until such evaluation is carried out and a complete perioperative care plan can be communicated with the surgical and anesthesia teams, so as to avoid bleeding complications.

Introduction

Von Willebrand disease (VWD) was first described in 1926 by a Finnish physician, Erik Adolf von Willebrand, after encountering a 5-year-old girl with history of bleeding [1]. VWD is identified as a quantitative or functional defect of the von Willebrand factor (VWF). The von Willebrand protein, commonly referred to as von Willebrand antigen (VWF:Ag), plays essential roles in platelet activation and adhesion in primary hemostasis. It is also a chaperone protein for factor VIII (FVIII), stabilizing the FVIII and prolonging its circulating half-life four–sixfold [2]. The incidence of VWD varies between 0.8% and 1.3% [3].

Clinical Presentation

VWD is typically an abnormality of the primary hemostatic pathway. Patients often present with skin- and mucosal lining-related bleeding: epistaxis, gum and oral bleeding (prolonged bleeding after tooth extractions and from biting the cheek or lips, and mouth bleeding), easy bruising, gastrointestinal tract bleeding, and/or menorrhagia. The presentation can vary based on the severity and type of disease.

There are many clinical variants of VWD, and the broad categorization is into three types: 1, 2, and 3. Type 1 is the commonest of the types of VWD and is a quantitative insufficiency of VWF:Ag. This chapter will focus on type 1 disease. Type 2 is a qualitative defect of the VWF:Ag, whereas type 3 indicates negligible to no circulating VWF.

Type 1 VWD Pathophysiology

Type 1 VWD accounts for about 75% of all VWD cases [4]. It is primarily inherited in an autosomal dominant pattern and is a partial deficiency of otherwise normal and functional VWF. Severity of symptoms in type 1 VWD typically correlates with degree of deficiency of the factor. Type 1 VWD, hence, can further be subclassified based on the degree of quantitative deficiency of VWF:Ag. VWD is an inheritable bleeding disorder with its genetic basis being much better understood now, due to advances over the last four decades.

The von Willebrand (VW) protein is a large glycoprotein produced in endothelial cells and bone marrow megakaryocytes. Its production includes sophisticated processes involving initial synthesis, dimerization, glycosylation, and then multimerization, packaging for storage and subsequently cleaving, and release into circulation for its function (Fig. 9.1). The VW protein has excess of 2800 amino acids. The gene controlling this execution is the *VWF* gene, on short arm of chromosome 12, which is 178 kb and made up of 52 codons [5]. The mature VW

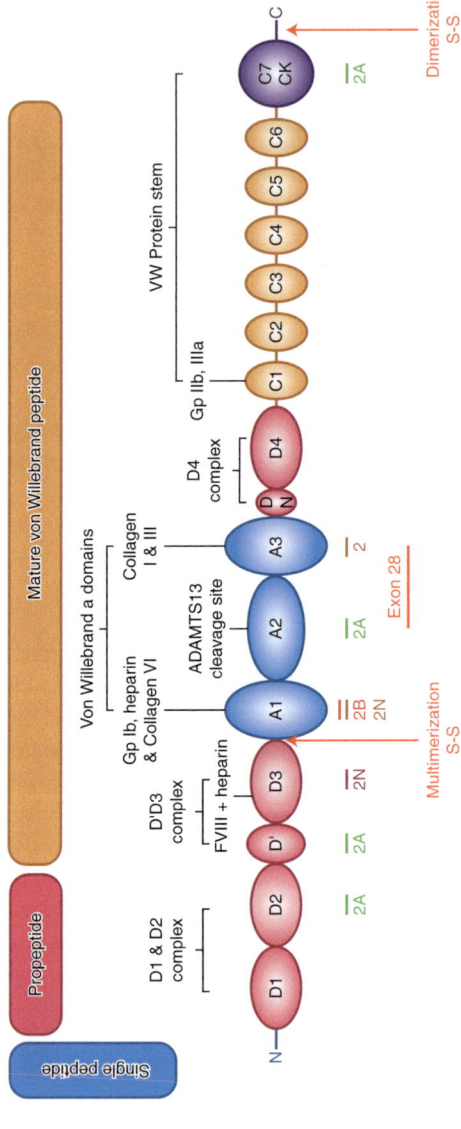

Fig. 9.1 Structure of the von Willebrand protein with binding sites and sites of qualitative defects

protein is stored in the alpha granules of platelets and the Weibel-Palade (WP) bodies of the endothelial cells in vessel wall lining. The defects leading to VWD occur at many steps during this processing of the peptide. The majority of type 1 VWD is due to missense mutations in the coding regions, promoter, or splice sites in the *VWF* gene [6].

The VWF protein, at baseline, circulates in a globular form and as a non-covalent complex with FVIII. Its activity is through two functions: first, it promotes hemostasis by mediating platelet adhesion to damaged vascular subendothelial matrix (e.g., collagen) and further platelet aggregation; second, it is the carrier protein for FVIII, protecting it from rapid proteolysis. The adhesive activity of VWF depends on the size of its multimers, with larger multimers being the most hemostatic. When there is exposure of sub-endothelium and modified flow dynamics with a vascular injury, a conformal change occurs in the VWF protein. As a result, the higher-molecular-weight multimers interact with collagen and platelet receptors with eventual regulatory participation from FVIII as well as in thrombus generation [7].

Besides vascular injury, there are a number of factors that can affect the circulating levels of VWF. Physiologically, the production of VWF in the body increases with age [8]. Also, pregnancy and high estrogen states can lead to increased VWF. Another hormonal pathway that can have an effect on VWF levels is thyroid, as hypothyroidism is associated with VWD. Stressors, such as a recent procedure or agitation due to blood draw, can increase the amount of VWF in the blood. A recent infection, inflammatory state, or anemia can also elevate VWF levels. Rigorous physical activity and exercise are known to raise the VWF level in the blood as well [9]. ABO blood groups can also exert a biological effect on VWF. People with type O blood have about 25% lower levels of VWF than people in blood groups A, B, and AB [10].

Type 1 Subclassification

Type 1 C – or "clearance type" – is a variant of type 1 VWD in which the survival of VWF is decreased due to increased clearance of the protein. It is also inherited in an autosomal dominant fashion and has another subtype known as the VWD Vicenza variant. The Vicenza-type VWD was originally described in patients from the Vicenza area in Italy and is notable for ultra-large multimers of VWF which are hypothesized to be subsequently cleared out of circulation, leaving behind very low level of plasma VWF despite the normal level of platelet VWF content [11].

Severe type 1 VWD is the quantitative deficiency of VWF, wherein significant clinical manifestations of bleeding may be present and can be seen at VWF:Ag and activity levels lower than 5 or 10 IU/dL. These patients usually have a correspondingly low FVIII, typically <20 IU/dL.

Differential Diagnosis

For patients presenting with mucocutaneous bleeding, consistent with a primary hemostatic-like defect, one must consider VWD in the differential. A detailed history and review of symptoms can help guide clinicians toward the diagnosis. To aid such history taking, multiple bleeding assessment tools have been designed, that help in screening patients for possible inherited bleeding diatheses. Several of these have been validated for VWD, namely, Vicenza bleeding score, the Pediatric Bleeding Questionnaire (PBQ), and ISTH/SSC Joint Working Group's Bleeding Assessment Tool (ISTH-BAT), including their self-administrable versions, the Self-BAT and Self-PBQ [12]. The exact cutoffs for bleeding score obtained from these tools vary based on the type of instrument and patient's age and gender, and continue to be an area of research. One may extrapolate from all these data that a score ≥ 2 can be considered abnormal for children [13] and can support initiating further workup for VWD.

Most bleeding assessment tools do not review the family history information. Hence, with a negative personal bleeding symptomatology, especially in the evaluation of children with none to minimal history of hemostatic challenges, family history is indispensable. If there is a known history of VWD or significant mucocutaneous bleeding in a close family member, it may be reasonable to proceed with initial evaluation, even with a low to normal patient bleeding score.

The differential for VWD includes abnormalities in platelet number, function- or adhesion-related defects, or dysfunction of collagen-platelet interaction. A quantitative defect of platelets, like immune thrombocytopenia, would also present in a similar bleeding phenotype. Disorders of collagen that interfere with platelet adhesion to sub-endothelium, e.g., Ehlers-Danlos syndrome, could also be difficult to discern from VWD in presentation.

Laboratory Findings

The evaluation for a bleeding disorder concerning for possible VWD, should start with a complete blood count (CBC). CBC can identify thrombocytopenia and other cellular abnormalities. Prothrombin time (PT) and partial thromboplastin time (PTT) are typically normal in VWD and can be part of the screen. In certain situations, PTT maybe prolonged, if the FVIII levels are low [14].

Platelet function analysis (PFA) can also detect more severe forms of VWD. It utilizes blood flowing through two different cartridges (containing either collagen plus ADP or collagen plus epinephrine). This test mimics the in vivo shear forces and activation of platelets followed by interaction with VWF, leading to hemostasis via clot/occlusion formation. In VWD, the PFA will be prolonged in both cartridges. Other platelet function issues can also give the same result though. Hence, prolonged PFA results are consistent with, but not specific for, VWD.

More specific testing for VWD to differentiate different subtypes, includes measurement of the von Willebrand protein itself (Table 9.1). This is achieved by carrying out an ELISA-based assay of the VWF:Ag and measurement of its function. The quantification of the VWF function is most commonly achieved by stimulating the platelet binding through use of antibiotic ristocetin as a cofactor [15]. The ristocetin-based testing for the VW function (VWF:RCo) can have high variability – in between different laboratories and within the same lab or same patients' sam-

Table 9.1 A table comparing inherited VWD types and its differential diagnosis. (Used with permission from John Wiley and Sons, from source: Nichols, W.L., Hultin, M.B., James, A.H., Manco-Johnson, M.J., Montgomery, R.R., Ortel, T.L., Rick, M.E., Sadler, J.E., Weinstein, M. and Yawn, B.P. (2008), von Willebrand disease (VWD): evidence-based diagnosis and management guidelines, the National Heart, Lung, and Blood Institute (NHLBI) Expert Panel report (USA) 1. Haemophilia, 14:171–232. https://doi.org/10.1111/j.1365-2516.2007.01643.x. This article is based on a U.S. government publication which is in the public domain.)

Disease type	Genetic transmission	VWF antigen (VWF:Ag)	VWF activity – ristocetin based (RCo)	VWF activity – GPIbM	Factor VIII level	VWF collagen binding assay (VWF:CB)	Multimer pattern	DDAVP responsiveness	Bleeding tendency	Frequency
1	Autosomal dominant	↓	↓	↓	↓	N or ↓	Normal	Good	Asymptomatic to moderately severe	70
2A	Autosomal dominant or recessive	N or ↓	N or ↓	N or ↓	N or ↓	↓↓↓	High and intermediate MW missing	Mild to moderate	Moderate to moderately severe	10–15
2B	Autosomal dominant	N or ↓	N or ↓	N or ↓	N or ↓	↓↓↓	High MW missing	DDAVP not indicated	Moderate to moderately severe	<5
2M	Autosomal dominant	N or ↓	↓ or ↓↓	N or ↓	N or ↓	Normal	Normal	Mild to moderate	Significant	10–15
2N	Autosomal recessive	Normal	Normal	Normal	↓ or ↓↓	Normal	Normal	Suboptimal	Mild to moderate	Uncommon
3	Autosomal recessive	↓↓↓	↓↓↓	↓↓↓	↓↓↓	↓↓↓	All multimers absent	No response	Severe	Rare
Platelet type VWD	Autosomal dominant	N or ↓	↓↓	N or ↓	N or ↓	Normal	High MW often missing	DDAVP not indicated	Moderate to moderately severe	Uncommon
D1472H/ p1467s	Autosomal recessive	Normal	↓	Normal	Normal	Normal	Normal	No clinical bleeding	None reported	Low

ples as well. It also does not directly measure physiologic function and is an indirect stimulator of VWF activity. Newer methodologies may prove more consistent and reliable. One of these is the glycoprotein IbM (GPIbM) testing, which utilizes a gain of function mutation-based assay, allowing the VWF to bind to platelets spontaneously, without needing ristocetin stimulation [16]. This assay is now commercially available from at least one reference laboratory in the United States. Factor VIII quantitative level is an important supplement to VWF functional evaluation, because it assesses the VWF's ability to bind to FVIII, preventing its proteolysis. FVIII level is important in differentiating the type 2 subtypes and for diagnosis of type 3 VWD.

Testing of the VWF multimers is another specific test for VWD, but the multimer distribution is typically normal in type 1 VWD (Fig. 9.2). When the VWF:Ag and VWF:RCo are both reduced in a proportionate fashion, multimer testing is not required, unless the clinician has concerns for type 2M disease. Platelet function and multimer evaluation are expanded upon further in the following chapter, as platelet testing is essential for variants of VWD type 2. More details on genetic testing for VWD are provided in Chapter 10.

With regard to the VWF:Ag and VWF:RCo testing, what levels should be considered diagnostic for VWD continues to be a matter of debate. The United Kingdom and National Heart, Lung, and Blood Institute (NHLBI) guidelines advise VWF:Ag and activity of less than 30 IU/dL, as being diagnostic of VWD. These define the range of 30–50 IU/dL to be "low von Willebrand levels", as patients in these ranges may also be experiencing symptoms that are more than the general population, but not severe enough to be called as disease [9, 17]. Canadian centers approach the diagnostic levels slightly differently and define levels <40 IU/dL as VWD. Per the NHLBI guidelines, those with low VWF levels, but a significant bleeding phenotype, may still be candidates for similar management as for those with VWD. For type 1C, the quantification of VWF propeptide can be helpful in making the correct diagnosis. There will be a higher circulating propeptide level than the VWF:Ag in type 1C.

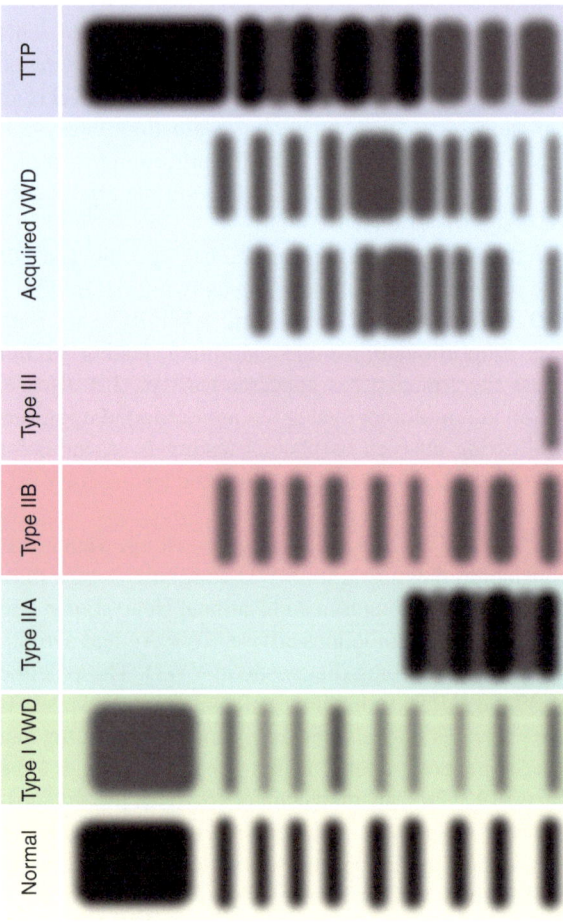

Fig. 9.2 Multimer distribution patterns in various von Willebrand disease forms. VWD von Willebrand disease, TTP thrombotic thrombocytopenic purpura. (Used with permission from source: Richard Torres, Yuri Fedoriw. *Laboratory Testing for von Willebrand Disease: Toward a Mechanism-Based Classification*, Clinics in Laboratory Medicine, 2009-06-01, Volume 29, Issue 2, Pages 193–228, Copyright © 2009 Elsevier Inc.)

> For our patient in the clinical case, with ristocetin cofactor level of 25% and a von Willebrand antigen level of 27%, a diagnosis of type 1 disease could be made. Multimer testing is not necessary for type 1 disease, and this can be determined by noting that the VWF activity and antigen levels are proportionately decreased (i.e., VW activity/antigen ratio is >0.6).

During the initial workup for VWD, one must remain cautious of all the factors and stressors that can transiently increase the levels of VWF as discussed earlier. Patients with blood type O are known to have lower VWF levels but may accordingly have bleeding phenotypes correlating well with their levels. Also, when approaching the decision on timing of testing, age and recent stressors should be taken into account. In young children and infants with strong family history of VWD, timing of testing can be challenging. Testing and any elective major hemostatic challenges should be delayed beyond 6 months to a year of age, when better quantification of innate VWF can be done.

Management Options

The management of VWD varies significantly with the type and severity of disease. The management options include (1) replacement therapy, (2) supportive and adjunctive therapies, and (3) anticipatory guidance to minimize bleeding complications in patients.

Replacement Factors

Replacement products are utilized with a goal of improving circulating levels of VWF and FVIII. Humate-P™, Alphanate™, and Wilate™ are the plasma-derived products approved by Food and Drug Administration (FDA) for use for VWD in the United States. These products directly increase the circulating VWF and

FVIII levels. They should be dosed based on their labeled content of VWF:RCo units, because each product is different for the content ratio of VWF:FVIII. Vonvendi™, the first recombinant VWD concentrate available in the United States, does not contain FVIII. It is not yet FDA approved for use in children.

Adjunctive Therapies

Desmopressin/DDAVP Desmopressin or 1-deamino-8-D-arginine vasopressin (DDAVP), is a synthetic vasopressin analogue that leads to release of VWF and subsequently increased plasma VWF and FVIII concentrations. It acts as an agonist at the V2 receptors in the WP bodies and has no effect on the platelet-stored VWF.

Its successful use requires an evaluation of the patient's ability to respond to it. Responsiveness is determined by "DDAVP challenge" testing. The challenge testing can be done with intranasal (IN) or intravenous (IV) DDAVP. Stimate® is the only brand of IN DDAVP that has sufficient concentration for VWD use. Young children (<5 years of age), who are unable to sniff on command, may be candidates for responsiveness testing through IV dosing. A baseline level of VWF:Ag and activity (RCo or GPIbM) and FVIII is obtained, followed by DDAVP administration. Then 1-, 2-, and 4-hour post levels are assessed to determine response. Successful response criteria include at least a twofold rise in VWF:Ag and VWF:RCo, in addition to achieving levels >30 IU/ml. In patients who do respond, if used too frequently, the response may wane once stored VWF is depleted. The most commonly studied frequency of use is every 24 hours for 3–4 doses. DDAVP should not be used any more than every 12 hours [9]. When used more frequently, tachyphylaxis may occur, and there is increasing risk of electrolyte disturbances. DDAVP's side-effect profile includes flushing, tachycardia, edema, and headache. DDAVP leads to water retention, which can result in hyponatremia and, subsequently, seizures. Careful anticipatory guidance about fluid intake is essential to limit side effects. A guide for the allowable fluid volumes for weight is provided in Table 9.2.

Table 9.2 Hydration guide for fluid intake after DDAVP use

Weight of the patient		Maximum fluid intake range for 24 hours after each DDAVP dose[a]	
Pounds	Kilograms	¾ Maintenance	Maintenance
<23	<10	Individualized per physician staff	
22–34	10–15	750 ml (25 ounces)	1000 ml (34 ounces)
35–45	16–20	975 ml (33 ounces)	1300 ml (44 ounces)
46–55	21–25	1140 ml (39 ounces)	1520 ml (51 ounces)
56–66	26–30	1215 ml (41 ounces)	1620 ml (55 ounces)
67–77	31–35	1290 ml (44 ounces)	1720 ml (58 ounces)
78–88	36–40	1365 ml (46 ounces)	1820 ml (62 ounces)
89–99	41–45	1440 ml (49 ounces)	1920 ml (65 ounces)
100–110	46–50	1515 ml (51 ounces)	2020 ml (68 ounces)
111–121	51–55	1590 ml (54 ounces)	2120 ml (72 ounces)
122–132	56–60	1665 ml (56 ounces)	2220 ml (75 ounces)
133–143	61–65	1740 ml (59 ounces)	2320 ml (78 ounces)
≥144–154	≥66–70	1800 ml (61 ounces)	2400 ml (81 ounces)

[a]Volumes are approximate

Patients with history of severe headaches/migraines, autonomic dysfunction, and seizures may do poorly due to the side-effect profile of DDAVP, and careful counseling and risk-benefit discussion should be carried out with the family before the test.

Additionally, DDAVP is contraindicated in some type 2 variants of VWD (discussed in further detail in Chapter 10). In type 1C, a transient increase in the VWF levels is seen at the 1-hour post DDAVP dose testing, but the 4-hour post level is again low.

Antifibrinolytics Synthetic lysine analogues, epsilon aminocaproic acid (EACA) and tranexamic acid (TXA), are agents that can be useful in stabilizing the fibrin clot in patients with defective hemostasis. They prevent fibrinolysis by inhibiting plasminogen activation. In bleeding from sites with higher concentration of natural fibrinolytics (e.g., nose, oropharynx, gastrointestinal tract), these prove effective in reducing clot breakdown. They can be used alone or as adjunctive therapy, with DDAVP or VWD concentrates.

EACA is available in a liquid formulation and pill form, but its high cost may prove prohibitive. TXA, on the other hand, is relatively cheaper but is only available in tablet form, which limits use in children. Both of these agents are available in injectable forms, for use in the perioperative and inpatient setting.

Other management approaches for specific bleeding manifestations in VWD (e.g., menorrhagia) are discussed in Chapter 10.

Comprehensive Care

VWD is a chronic condition that can affect many facets of the lives of patients. For patients with significant bleeding symptoms, quality of life can be poor as their symptoms may pose several limitations on their activities. Patients with VWD should be cared for in hemophilia treatment centers (HTCs). HTCs offer comprehensive care with multidisciplinary expertise. These centers have specialized experience in guiding the management of complicated scenarios like surgeries, trauma-related bleeding, access to research protocols, as well as newer developments in the management of bleeding disorders. Annual to biannual comprehensive visits, based on the frequency of bleeding symptoms, can help improve the general health maintenance for children with VWD.

Clinical Pearls and Pitfalls
- Mucosal bleeding is the most common manifestation of von Willebrand disease.
- Glycoprotein IbM testing is an alternative to ristocetin cofactor testing to measure von Willebrand factor activity.
- Desmopressin affects fluid balance; thus, careful anticipatory guidance on fluid intake is essential to avoid side effects.
- Stimate is the only brand of intranasal DDAVP appropriate for use in VWD.
- Antifibrinolytic agents are a useful adjunctive therapy.

- Von Willebrand levels can be affected by stress, exercise, and inflammation, so testing results should be interpreted with caution in these settings.
- Patients who are pregnant or on estrogen-containing medications may have higher than baseline VW levels due to the estrogen effect.

References

1. Von Willebrand E. Hereditary pseudohemofilia. Fin Lakaresallsk Handl. 1926;68:87–112.
2. Lenting PJ, VAN Schooten CJ, Denis CV. Clearance mechanisms of von Willebrand factor and factor VIII. J Thromb Haemost. 2007;5(7):1353–60.
3. Werner EJ, Broxson EH, Tucker EL, Giroux DS, Shults J, Abshire TC. Prevalence of von Willebrand disease in children: a multiethnic study. J Pediatr. 1993;123(6):893–8.
4. Haberichter SL, Castaman G, Budde U, Peake I, Goodeve A, Rodeghiero F, et al. Identification of type 1 von Willebrand disease patients with reduced von Willebrand factor survival by assay of the VWF propeptide in the European study: molecular and clinical markers for the diagnosis and management of type 1 VWD (MCMDM-1VWD). Blood. 2008;111(10):4979–85.
5. Sadler JE. Biochemistry and genetics of von Willebrand factor. Annu Rev Biochem. 1998;67:395–424.
6. Lillicrap D. Genotype/phenotype association in von Willebrand disease: is the glass half full or empty? J Thromb Haemost. 2009;7(Suppl 1):65–70.
7. Wagner DD. Cell biology of von Willebrand factor. Annu Rev Cell Biol. 1990;6:217–46.
8. Sanders YV, Giezenaar MA, Laros-van Gorkom BA, Meijer K, van der Bom JG, Cnossen MH, et al. von Willebrand disease and aging: an evolving phenotype. J Thromb Haemost. 2014;12(7):1066–75.
9. Nichols WL, Hultin MB, James AH. Von Willebrand disease (VWD): evidence- based diagnosis and management guidelines, the National Heart, Lung, and Blood Institute (NHLBI) expert panel report (USA). Haemophilia. 2008;14:171–232.
10. Jenkins PV, O'Donnell JS. ABO blood group determines plasma von Willebrand factor levels: a biologic function after all? Transfusion. 2006;46(10):1836–44.

11. Mannucci PM, Lombardi R, Castaman G, Dent JA, Lattuada A, Rodeghiero F, et al. von Willebrand disease "Vicenza" with larger-than-normal (supranormal) von Willebrand factor multimers. Blood. 1988;71(1):65–70.
12. Bowman ML, James PD. Bleeding scores for the diagnosis of von Willebrand disease. Semin Thromb Hemost. 2017;43(5):530–9.
13. O'Brien SH. Bleeding scores: are they really useful? Hematology Am Soc Hematol Educ Program. 2012;2012:152–6.
14. Castaman G, Rodeghiero F. Advances in the diagnosis and management of type 1 von Willebrand disease. Expert Rev Hematol. 2011;4(1):95–106.
15. Vanhoorelbeke K, Cauwenberghs N, Vauterin S, Schlammadinger A, Mazurier C, Deckmyn H. A reliable and reproducible ELISA method to measure ristocetin cofactor activity of von Willebrand factor. Thromb Haemost. 2000;83(1):107–13.
16. Sharma R, Flood VH. Advances in the diagnosis and treatment of Von Willebrand disease. Blood. 2017;130(22):2386–91.
17. Laffan MA, Lester W, O'Donnell JS, Will A, Tait RC, Goodeve A, et al. The diagnosis and management of von Willebrand disease: a United Kingdom Haemophilia Centre Doctors Organization guideline approved by the British Committee for Standards in Haematology. Br J Haematol. 2014;167(4):453–65.

Presentation and Management of Type 2 von Willebrand Disease

Dominder Kaur and Sarah H. O'Brien

10

Case Presentation A 16-year-old female with history of hematochezia and melena was sent to you by gastroenterology, for evaluation of a possible bleeding disorder. Patient denies recent constipation, diarrhea, vomiting, or abdominal/rectal pain. On detailed history, you also identify complaints of easy bruising and past report of heavy menstrual periods, but the latter have improved since her gynecologist started her on oral contraceptive pills. Her labs show a normal CBC, normal PT and PTT, a mildly prolonged platelet func-

D. Kaur (✉)
Department of Pediatrics, Division of Pediatric Hematology/Oncology/Stem Cell Transplant, Columbia University Irving Medical Center, Children's Hospital of New York/New York Presbyterian Morgan Stanley Children's Hospital, New York, NY, USA
e-mail: dk3076@cumc.columbia.edu

S. H. O'Brien
Nationwide Children's Hospital, Division of Pediatric Hematology, Oncology and Bone Marrow Transplant, Columbus, OH, USA

Center for Innovation in Pediatric Practice, Abigail Wexner Research Institute at Nationwide Children's Hospital, Columbus, OH, USA

Department of Pediatrics, The Ohio State University College of Medicine, Columbus, OH, USA
e-mail: Sarah.Obrien@nationwidechildrens.org

© Springer Nature Switzerland AG 2020
A. L. Dunn et al. (eds.), *Pediatric Bleeding Disorders*,
https://doi.org/10.1007/978-3-030-31661-7_10

tion analysis (PFA), and von Willebrand antigen of 44% but ristocetin cofactor activity of 25%. Multimer evaluation was sent out and revealed loss of high-molecular-weight (HMW) multimers.

Management

This diagnosis is consistent with von Willebrand disease (VWD) type 2A. The likely etiology for her bloody stools is:

(a) Mallory-Weiss tear
(b) Gastroenteritis-related bleeding that was exacerbated by her type 2A VWD
(c) **Angiodysplasia in the gastrointestinal (GI) lining**
(d) Intussusception, as it is a common occurrence in VWD type 2A

> Mucosal bleeding is the most common type of bleeding seen in patients with von Willebrand disease. With regard to the etiology of bloody stools, gastrointestinal (GI) angiodysplasia is more likely than the other possibilities. Intussusception is not a common occurrence in type 2A patients. GI bleeding is relatively common in patients with type 2 VWD, and this patient does not have symptoms of gastroenteritis.

Clinical Presentation, Classification, and Pathophysiology

Type 2 von Willebrand disease (VWD) is a group of primary hemostatic defects, which present primarily with mucocutaneous bleeding including epistaxis, GI tract bleeding, and menorrhagia. It has four clinical subtypes (2A, 2B, 2M, 2N) caused by qualitative defects in the von Willebrand factor (VWF) protein. This is in contrast to type 1 and 3 VWD, which are quantitative defects. Type 2 VWD is inherited in an autosomal dominant fashion except for type 2N, which is inherited recessively. The bleeding symptoms are often intermediate between that of milder type 1 disease and the more severe type 3 disease. A personal history of bleeding events and a detailed family history can help guide clinicians toward the diagnosis.

VWD Type 2A

Type 2A VWD is the commonest of the type 2 variants [1]. It is characterized by preferential loss of the large- and intermediate-molecular-weight (MW) multimers, leading to defective platelet binding. Multiple etiologies are postulated for this loss of the high MW multimers – with several causative mutations having been identified. The most common mutation in type 2A is one that renders the protein more susceptible to proteolysis by ADAMTS13. There are other mutations that interfere with multimerization or assembly after multimer production. A large majority of the missense mutations are in the exon 28 region of the *VWF* gene in the A2 domain, whereas a minority affect the A1 domain. Additional multimerization defects via mutations in propeptide or N-terminus regions or dimerization defects with CK terminus mutations are also reported [2].

VWD Type 2B

Type 2B is a gain-of-function phenotype of VWD, characterized by increased binding of platelets. It is most commonly caused by missense mutations in the A1 domain of VWF gene exon 28, which enhance the binding of VWF to platelet receptor glycoprotein Ibα (GpIbα). Because of the increased binding, more platelet-VWF complexes circulate in the plasma and subsequently, undergo proteolytic degradation by ADAMTS13. Result is a lower number of platelets and depletion of the high MW multimers of VWF. It is also reported that the remaining platelets may be less functional, because of having VWF bound on them [3].

An opposite gain-of-function property on the platelet surface, leading to increased binding of VWF onto platelets, leads to another variant of the disease known as platelet-type VWD.

VWD Type 2M

Type 2M ("M"ultimerically normal) VWD is associated with a loss of function mutation, in contrast to the gain-of-function mutations in 2B. There are two main causes of 2M VWD. The first is caused by a defect in binding to Gp1bα leading to inadequate platelet adhesion. This is caused by missense mutations in the A1 domain. A second type of 2M is linked with mutations in the A3 domain and is associated with defective VWF interaction with collagen. The multimers are normally distributed in 2M disease, and mutation analysis is useful for confirming a diagnosis.

VWD Type 2N

VWD 2N is named after "Normandy" where the first individuals with this subtype were identified; they were noted to have decreased FVIII due to VWF defects of FVIII binding. The presentation is very similar to hemophilia A, and often these patients can initially be misdiagnosed as having hemophilia. As opposed to type 1 and other subtypes of type 2 VWD, there can be spontaneous bleeding into joints and muscles and large hematoma formation with minor trauma in VWD 2N. The family history is helpful in those scenarios as type 2N is inherited in an autosomal recessive fashion and can occur in women. A genetic mutation analysis and/or VWF to FVIII binding assay can confirm the diagnosis. The mutations in type 2N commonly occur in the hypermutable arginine codons in domain D or the FVIII binding region of VWF. The levels of FVIII may be in the mild-to-moderate deficiency ranges, based on the degree of poor binding with VWF, and often <10–20%. The VWF antigen and activity may be proportionately reduced and can also be low to normal in type 2N disease, along with a normal multimer distribution pattern.

Differential Diagnosis

The differential diagnosis of type 2 VWD is similar to type 1 disease, especially as presenting symptoms are of bleeding from mucosal surfaces. The differential diagnosis includes conditions with quantitative platelet defects, e.g., immune thrombocytopenia (ITP) or qualitative platelet dysfunction like Bernard-Soulier syndrome, Glanzmann's thrombasthenia, or platelet storage pool deficiency. Inheritable collagen disorders like Ehlers-Danlos syndrome can also present with skin and mucosal bleeding.

Type 2B-related thrombocytopenia can be misdiagnosed as chronic ITP in some cases. In addition, type 2B and platelet-type VWD are difficult to differentiate because of very similar presentation and pathophysiology. The platelet-type VWD is actually a defect on the platelet receptor GpIb, instead of on the VWF protein – that still leads to increased binding of VWF and platelets, leading to elimination of the platelet-VWF complexes and loss of high MW multimers.

Type 2N disease can often be misdiagnosed as hemophilia A because of the decrease in FVIII levels.

Laboratory Findings

The diagnosis of VWD should be suspected when a patient presents with history of mucocutaneous bleeding, especially if there is a positive family history. Type 2 VWD is likely when quantitative level of VWF:Ag is noted to be normal to low, but VWF structure and/or function is defective (Fig. 10.1).

Initial laboratory evaluation should include complete blood counts (CBC), prothrombin time, activated partial thromboplastin time, and von Willebrand antigen and activity levels. The von Willebrand activity to antigen ratio is helpful in identifying the functional defect of type 2 VWD. An activity to antigen ratio (or ristocetin cofactor activity to VWF:Ag ratio) of <0.6 indicates that the antigen is present but likely dysfunctional (Fig. 10.2).

Multimer pattern analysis is helpful in differentiating the various type 2 subtypes. It is carried out via electrophoresis in agarose gel and allows for visualization of the multimers (Fig. 9.2). The distribution shows loss of the large and intermediate multimers (the high-molecular-weight multimers) in types 2A and 2B and in platelet-type VWD. In type 2B, satellite banding may also be seen, from increased proteolytic degradation products out of the HMW multimers via ADAMTS13. Typically in type 1 VWD, the

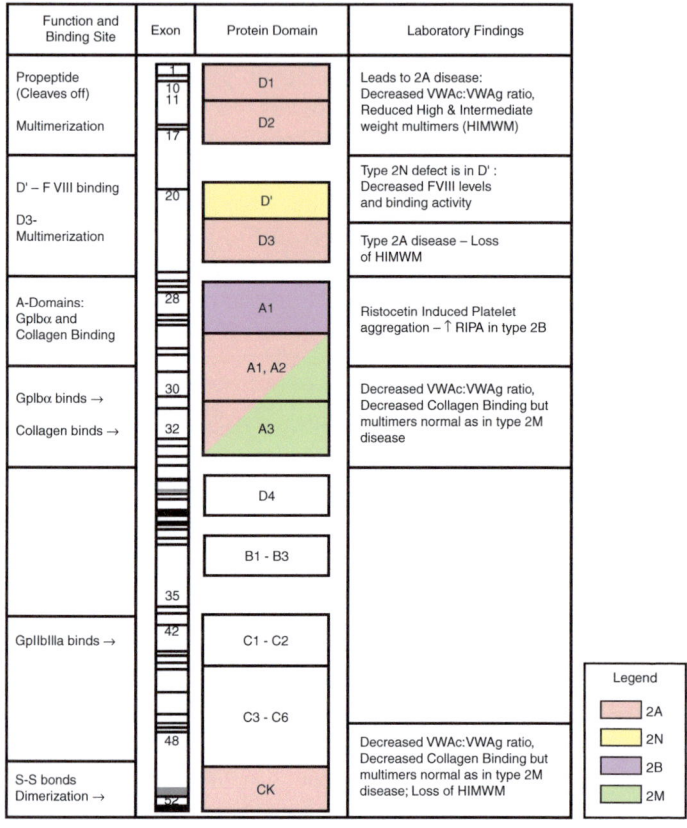

Fig. 10.1 Von Willebrand factor protein structure, functional sites, and laboratory findings. FVIII = factor VIII, VWAc = VWF activity, VWAg = VWF antigen, RCo = ristocetin cofactor, HIMWM = high- and intermediate-molecular-weight multimers, S-S = disulfide bonds, FVIII:B = factor VIII binding assay, VWF:CB = VWF collagen binding assay, RIPA = ristocetin-induced platelet aggregation, GpIbα = glycoprotein Ibα, GpIIb/IIIa = glycoprotein IIb/IIIa

multimeric distribution is normal, with the Vicenza variant being an exception (wherein ultralarge VWF multimers may be seen but low VWF).

The best approach to testing von Willebrand activity is debatable. The VWF:RCo assay is the most commonly used and widely available assay, but has many limitations. Ristocetin is a non-

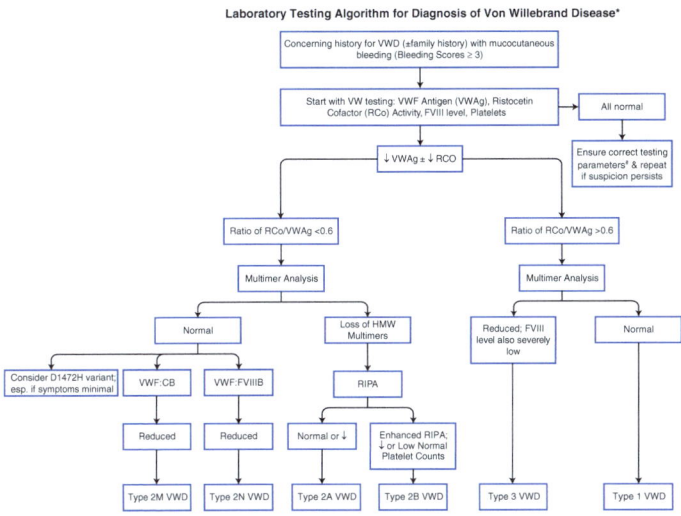

Fig. 10.2 Laboratory evaluation algorithm in VWD. VWD von Willebrand disease, VWAg VWF antigen, RCo ristocetin cofactor, RIPA ristocetin-induced platelet aggregation, FVIII factor VIII, FVIII:B factor VIII binding assay, VWF:CB VWF collagen binding assay. *Correct testing parameters may mean many different factors like timing of testing, sample handling and transport, ensuring blood draw without significant agitation and struggle to find a vein, and not testing a female who is on estrogen therapy

physiological agonist, and the VWF may bind to it variably, which can affect results [4]. This high coefficient of variability and binding difficulty becomes more pronounced when the VWF levels are low, around 10–20 IU/dL, making the same its lower limit of detection.

A newer assay to study VWF function, that utilizes gain-of-function modification of platelet GpIbα, has been developed. This is called the GpIbM assay. It allows for greater precision and can assess activity at VWF levels as low as 2 IU/dL. It is available commercially in automated versions in Canada and Europe, but availability is currently limited in the United States [5]. GpIbM assay will detect the lower functional activity in type 2A and shows reduced to normal activity for types 2B, 2M, and 2N. Another functional assay is the collagen binding assay; this is ELISA based and evaluates the ability of VWF to bind collagen. It is often seen as a supplementary test to the VWF:RCo. It also is abnormal (reduced) for types 2A, 2B, and 2M but is normal in type 2N.

One additional test that can be helpful in separating out the type 2 subtypes, is the ristocetin-induced platelet aggregation (RIPA) or low-dose RIPA (LD-RIPA). It is especially helpful in differentiating types 2A and 2B, if the platelet count is normal. The test is carried out by creating a low concentration of ristocetin in platelet-rich plasma. The low-dose ristocetin is not sufficient to lead to binding and aggregation of normal plasma and other types of VWD, but leads to aggregation in VWD 2B and platelet-type VWD. A similar test, that is donor platelet based, is helpful in differentiating platelet-type VWD from type 2B VWD. This is called the platelet binding assay.

Genetic testing is increasingly useful in diagnosis of type 2 disease and is perhaps more readily available than some of the more specialized testing mentioned above. It is often helpful in differentiating type 2N from mild hemophilia and hemophilia carrier states. It can also identify the correct diagnosis when phenotypic testing proves inconclusive. The common important mutations seen in types 2A, 2B, and 2M are located in exon 28, and limited exon testing can thus be carried out [6]. Exon 28 testing can aid the correct diagnosis when VWF activity to antigen ratio is decreased, but multimers are normal.

Importance of D1472H

An important genetic variant, that affects the ristocetin-cofactor-based activity assay of VWF, is important to consider when evaluating for type 2 VWD. The D1472H variant leads to significantly lower VWF:RCo activity and can cause spuriously low VWF:RCo/VWF:Ag ratios. It is more prevalent in the African-American population, but can also occur in Caucasians [7]. The finding is limited to testing that is ristocetin based. Other functional testing modalities, like collagen binding and the GpIbM assay, are not affected and reveal accurate VWF activity results. Patients with the D1472 variant do not have a true hemorrhagic risk, and thus, identifying this variant is helpful in preventing false diagnosis. Maintaining a high index of suspicion and obtaining appropriate functional testing like GpIbM assay and multimer analysis (which will be normal), can help in identifying this variant.

> With regard to our case, patient had a VWF activity to antigen ratio of <0.6 (25/44 = 0.56), indicating a functional von Willebrand defect. The low ratio was sufficient to warrant further evaluation for one of the type 2 variants, and hence, multimer testing was obtained. It revealed loss of large- and intermediate-sized multimers, which is characteristic of type 2A VWD.

Management Options

Topics for anticipatory guidance in patients with type 2 VWD include (1) bleed prevention, (2) supportive care (3), and treatment of specific bleeds.

To reduce the risk of bleeding, all patients with VWD should avoid nonsteroidal anti-inflammatory agents and anticoagulants. When regular use of NSAIDs is indicated (e.g., patients with chronic pain or arthritis), celecoxib is the preferred alternative because it is a selective cyclooxygenase 2 inhibitor with limited risk of bleeding [8]. Additionally, they should refrain from participation in high-risk activities and contact sports. They should also have individualized home and emergency department plans for minor and major bleeding events. Families should have ready access to supportive care measures like nose clips, ice packs, and compressive bandages. In select patients, home medication training and support including antifibrinolytic agents, factor replacement, or DDAVP should be considered.

DDAVP, a synthetic vasopressin analogue, can be used in some patients with type 2 disease. It is most commonly used in those with type 2A and 2M subtypes. It should only be utilized after documentation of a successful DDAVP challenge test. DDAVP can lead to increased platelet aggregation in type 2B and is relatively contraindicated. Cautions of fluid restriction (Table 9.2) while utilizing DDAVP should be exercised and education about the commonest side effects like headache, facial flushing, and dizziness provided to patients. Also, distinguishing the platelet-type VWD from type 2B is paramount, because VWF replacement therapy does not improve factor levels in this condition.

Antifibrinolytic agents – epsilon aminocaproic acid and tranexamic acid – can be used for bleeding management as these agents help stabilize the clots formed in patients with VWD.

For most minor procedures and injuries, the therapeutic goal should be to increase circulating VWF activity to approximately 50% of normal. For major surgeries or in situations with high bleeding risk, higher targets of 80–100% activity levels should be considered. The initial frequency of replacement factor dosing is every 6–12 hours and then, should be guided by bleeding symptoms and laboratory assessments. Typically, maintaining higher levels close to 100% for 2–4 days post major surgery or trauma and then, reducing frequency and targets to half for the next 7 days, followed by maintaining minor injury type targets (20–40 IU/dL) for the subsequent week, can be sufficient and provide adequate hemostasis (Tables 10.1 and 11.2).

Plasma-derived VWF concentrate products licensed for prophylaxis or bleeding events include Humate-P™, Wilate™, and Alphanate™. Among these, Humate-P™ has the highest VWF:RCo to FVIII content, but drug availability may be center dependent. A recombinant VWF concentrate without FVIII – Vonvendi™ – is now FDA approved for use in adults. Patients treated with this drug, who have concomitantly low FVIII levels, require addition of FVIII concentrate until the patients' own FVIII can be stabilized in circulation (takes 6–8 hours) or a pre-procedural initial dose should be provided to allow this time duration. Throughout replacement therapy, peak and trough monitoring may be helpful to ensure avoiding higher than 200–250% factor VIII levels and risk of thrombosis.

Table 10.1 Treatment approaches, products, and respective doses

Treatment approach and product		
Replacement therapies	**Dosage guide**[b]	**Dosing frequency**
Major bleeding/surgery	Loading dose 40–60 IU/kg[a] Maintenance: 20–40 IU/kg[a]	Every 8–24 hours based on invasiveness of procedure
Minor bleeding/procedures	Loading dose 30–60 IU/kg[a] Maintenance: 20–40 IU/kg[a]	Every 12–24 hours based on type of procedure and risk of bleeding
Adjunctive therapies		
DDAVP – IV DDAVP	0.3 micrograms/kg diluted in 25–50 mL normal saline infused over 30 minutes	Ideally every 24 hours for 3–4 doses (no more than every 12 hours – maximum three doses)
Intranasal DDAVP	150 micrograms (one puff) if ≤50 kg; 300 micrograms (two puffs) if >50 kg	
Aminocaproic acid	100–200 mg/kg P.O./IV loading; followed by 50–100 mg/kg/dose po/iv	Every 6 hours for 7–14 days
Tranexamic acid	(Only FDA approved for use in ≥12 years old) 1300 mg every 8 hours for up to 5 days	Every 8 hours for 7–10 days (up to 5 days for menorrhagia)

IU international units, *kg* kilograms, *DDAVP* desmopressin or 1-deamino-8-D-arginine vasopressin, *P.O.* per os/by mouth, *IV* intravenous, *FDA* Food and Drug Administration

[a]Based on RCO units in products

[b]Sample guidance. The clinical scenario and patient profile should be used to guide dosing and adjustments

Continuous infusions of VWF products can also be used in surgical and immediately postsurgical settings.

Management of selected bleeding events in non-DDAVP-responsive patients:

Bleeding from Gastrointestinal (GI) Tract

VWF is hypothesized to have a role in endothelial cell proliferation and angiogenesis due to its presence in the WP bodies of the endothelial cells. A common manifestation of this role is noted in GI tract angiodysplasia, that is prevalent in 2–4% patients with type 2 and 3 VWD. Within type 2, type 2A VWD (and less commonly type 2B), patients experience angiodysplasia-related GI bleeding. Dark-colored stools or fresh bleeding may both be seen. Antifibrinolytics can prove helpful in such settings. VWF replacement is indicated in patients with significant or ongoing blood loss.

Epistaxis

Patients should sit up with their head slightly forward and apply firm pressure at the base of the nasal bone for 10–20 minutes. Nasal ice packs and nose clips may also prove helpful. Vascular constrictive nasal sprays can be useful, but should not be used longer than 3 days in succession. Packing should be avoided, unless bleeding cannot be stopped with local measures. Antifibrinolytic therapy is typically helpful and should be continued for 24 hours after the cessation of bleeding. VWF concentrate targeting 50% VWF:RCo is indicated for persistent epistaxis. Patients who experience recurrent epistaxis, can consider topical use of estrogen cream [9]. Typical application cycle for this therapy can be daily at night (qHS) for 6 months, alternating with 6-months off therapy, to avoid any long-term effects and significant systemic absorption.

Menorrhagia

Adolescents and young adults with VWD commonly experience menorrhagia. It is frequently complicated by anemia and decreased quality of life. A multidisciplinary approach with adolescent medicine and/or gynecologic support in addition to the HTC support is optimal. Estrogen containing hormonal contraceptives are a mainstay of care, as these agents can increase the baseline VWF level in the patient with non-severe disease. Other progesterone-specific hormonal options may be helpful in regularizing or temporarily stopping the menstrual blood losses. Antifibrinolytics can be used alone or in combination with hormonal agents, but the risk of venous thromboembolic events should be considered. For more severe bleeding phenotypes or when other methodologies do not provide adequate hemostasis, therapy should include factor concentrates.

> *Management Question Response*: **Angiodysplasia in the Gastrointestinal Lining**
> The gastrointestinal bleeding could be managed initially with VWF concentrate with an initial major bleeding dose, with VWF: RCo correction of about 80% for the first day, followed by maintaining levels to ~50% for the subsequent 2–3 days. Once active hemorrhage is controlled, gastrointestinal consultation to identify extent of angiodysplasia is indicated. Typically, older patients show increasing degree of angiodysplasia and will have worse bleeding complications than young and pediatric patients. In this patient, as she has history of menorrhagia as well, as-needed use of DDAVP, may prove helpful.

Clinical Pearls and Pitfalls
- All type 2 von Willebrand variants are qualitative deficiencies of von Willebrand protein.
- A von Willebrand antigen to ristocetin cofactor ratio of <0.6 is indicative of type 2 disease.
- Mild-to-moderate thrombocytopenia in a patient with mucosal bleeding should prompt an evaluation for type 2B VWD (or platelet type VWD).
- Genetic testing can also prove quite helpful in clarifying equivocal or difficult cases.
- Angiodysplasia in the GI tract is a frequent complication of 2A disease.
- The majority of type 2 mutations occur within exon 28 of the VW gene.
- DDAVP is less likely to be effective in type 2 VWD compared to type 1.

References

1. Ng C, Motto DG, Di Paola J. Diagnostic approach to von Willebrand disease. Blood. 2015;125(13):2029–37.
2. Lillicrap D. Genotype/phenotype association in von Willebrand disease: is the glass half full or empty? J Thromb Haemost. 2009;7(Suppl 1):65–70.
3. Nichols WL, Hultin MB, James AH. Von Willebrand disease (VWD): evidence- based diagnosis and management guidelines, the National Heart, Lung, and Blood Institute (NHLBI) expert panel report (USA). Haemophilia. 2008;14:171–232.
4. Patzke J, Budde U, Huber A, Méndez A, Muth H, Obser T, et al. Performance evaluation and multicentre study of a von Willebrand factor activity assay based on GPIb binding in the absence of ristocetin. Blood Coagul Fibrinolysis. 2014;25(8):860–70.
5. Sharma R, Flood VH. Advances in the diagnosis and treatment of Von Willebrand disease. Blood. 2017;130(22):2386–91.
6. James PD, Goodeve AC. von Willebrand disease. Genet Med. 2011;13(5):365–76.
7. Flood VH, Gill JC, Morateck PA, Christopherson PA, Friedman KD, Haberichter SL, et al. Common VWF exon 28 polymorphisms in African Americans affecting the VWF activity assay by ristocetin cofactor. Blood. 2010;116(2):280–6.
8. Lie HK, Turner SC. Early experience with the use of celecoxib in a child and adolescent population. J Pharm Pract Res. 2002;32(1):27–31.
9. Ross CS, Pruthi RK, Schmidt KA, Eckerman AL, Rodriguez V. Intranasal oestrogen cream for the prevention of epistaxis in patients with bleeding disorders. Haemophilia. 2011;17(1):164.

Clinical Approach to Type 3 von Willebrand Disease

11

Dominder Kaur and Sarah H. O'Brien

Case Presentation You receive a call from the ED about a toddler being evaluated with oral bleeding. He was playing with his sister earlier this morning, when he fell and tore his frenulum. He has had easy bruising in the past. Parents report no known family history of bleeding disorders. They have not had him evaluated for the bruising because both parents have had similar type of bruising themselves and did not find it concerning. In the ED, his initial labs

---

D. Kaur (✉)
Department of Pediatrics, Division of Pediatric Hematology/Oncology/Stem Cell Transplant, Columbia University Irving Medical Center, Children's Hospital of New York/New York Presbyterian Morgan Stanley Children's Hospital, New York, NY, USA
e-mail: dk3076@cumc.columbia.edu

S. H. O'Brien
Nationwide Children's Hospital, Division of Pediatric Hematology, Oncology and Bone Marrow Transplant, Columbus, OH, USA

Center for Innovation in Pediatric Practice, Abigail Wexner Research Institute at Nationwide Children's Hospital, Columbus, OH, USA

Department of Pediatrics, The Ohio State University College of Medicine, Columbus, OH, USA
e-mail: Sarah.Obrien@nationwidechildrens.org

show a normal CBC, except for mild anemia with a hemoglobin of 10.6 g/dL, prolonged partial thromboplastin time (PTT) at 39 sec, and normal prothrombin time (PT). He is admitted to the hospital due to persistent bleeding, and additional testing reveals that his factor VIII (FVIII:C) and von Willebrand factor (VWF) levels are both less than 3 IU/dL. Repeat testing and multimer evaluation was sent and pending, with current working diagnosis of type 3 VWD. What is the appropriate therapy for him?

Multiple-Choice Management Question

(a) Intravenous DDAVP today followed by intranasal DDAVP Q48 hours for three doses
(b) Aminocaproic acid 50 mg/kg swish and swallow
(c) Factor VIII replacement; 20–40 IU/kg
(d) Replacement with von Willebrand factor and factor VIII-containing concentrates
(e) Oral surgery consultation
(f) **Both b and d**

Case Management

With the presumed diagnosis of type 3 VWD and ongoing bleeding, primary management will require replacement of the missing factors. In this quantitative defect of VWD, circulating factor VIII (FVIII) levels are also low, and accordingly, replacement will need to be with agents that contain both VWF and FVIII. Factor VIII replacement alone will not be successful in controlling bleeding because of its short (<20 minutes) half-life without VWF. DDAVP may be useful in type 1 VWD and some type 2 variants, but is not helpful in type 3. Antifibrinolytics can be useful adjuncts for mucosal bleeding.

Clinical Presentation

Type 3 VWD is characterized by total or near-total deficiency of VWF, with circulating VWF antigen and activity levels being less than 10% typically. It is the rarest form of VWD but may be the earliest form to be recognized, as onset of symptoms can occur as early as infancy. Patients with type 3 VWD can have more frequent and severe bleeding symptoms compared to other forms of this disease. Mucocutaneous bleeding is the most commonly seen symptom (nosebleeds, menstrual and postpartum hemorrhage, or gastrointestinal (GI) bleeding) followed by prolonged bleeding after surgical interventions or tooth extractions. Spontaneous bleeding in the form of muscle hematomas and joint bleeding can be seen in type 3 VWD and is thought to result from concomitant low FVIII levels. Rare instances of intracranial hemorrhage in neonates and children have also been reported [1].

Epidemiology and Inheritance

Among the types of von Willebrand disease, type 3 VWD is the rarest, making up less than 6% of all cases [2]. Its incidence is reported to be 0.5–1.4 per million, but higher incidence is noted in certain areas where consanguineous marriages are common [3]. Type 3 VWD is inherited as an autosomal recessive trait, with homozygous or composite heterozygous forms (with null alleles) being described. The causative genetic anomalies commonly reported are missense, frameshift and splice-site mutations, but large deletions in the VWF gene on 12p13.3 are also reported [4]. The overall result is synthesis of a truncated protein, that leads to negligible VWF levels or allele silencing.

The parents of patients with type 3 VWD or the heterozygous carriers of type 3 disease may or may not always provide a significant bleeding history. As the disease carriers have the autosomal recessive forms of type 3 VWD, in comparison with type 1

VWD carriers, bleeding symptoms are reportedly less frequent [5, 6]. Also, typically, the carriers of severe type 1 VWD may exhibit lower quantitative VWF levels than type 3 carriers, while some of the parents of type 3 VWD patients may not have any laboratory findings of VWF deficiency [4].

Differential Diagnosis

Being the chaperone protein for factor VIII, when circulating VWF is negligible to none, there is significant associated FVIII deficiency as well. Low FVIII levels are not a result of decreased synthesis of FVIII but due to increased proteolysis in the absence of the VWF chaperone protein. Because of this, type 3 VWD may present in a fashion very similar to hemophilia A (HA) and misdiagnosis as HA is a common mistake in type 3 VWD. Severe forms of type 2 variants and acquired VWD are the other forms of VWD that should be excluded. These variants need different therapeutic approaches; hence, correct diagnosis becomes essential. Vascular-type Ehlers-Danlos syndrome can also present with mucosal bleeding symptoms and joint subluxations/dislocations, but lack of physical findings such as joint and skin laxity and characteristic facial features would help exclude this diagnosis.

Laboratory Findings

Evaluation of type 3 VWD starts the same as most bleeding disorders and should include a complete blood count, prothrombin time (PT), partial thromboplastin time (PTT), fibrinogen, thrombin time (TT), and von Willebrand levels. Platelet count, PT, TT, and fibrinogen are normal in type 3 VWD. An elevated PTT and very low to nearly absent VW antigen and activity levels (1–9 IU/dL), along with a decreased FVIII activity assay, indicate likely type 3 VWD. Multimer testing will show absent to negligible protein, and no specific pattern in the distribution is discernible. Ristocetin-induced platelet aggregation is also reduced in this variant.

The diagnosis is made on primary labs but can be further supported with genetic testing findings. There are many types of mutations known to be associated with type 3 VWD and include nonsense, frameshift, splicing, missense substitutions, and exonic to large complete VWF gene deletions [3].

Another test, the VWF propeptide assay, can prove useful in differentiating type 3 disease from severe type 1 variants, especially the type 1C or "clearance" subtype. During its production in the body, VW protein consists of a signal peptide of 22 amino acids and a propeptide of 741 amino acids. The propeptide gets released from the VWF protein's precursor form as a cleavage product, before the mature protein is stored in the Weibel-Palade (WP) bodies. In severe type 1 disease/type 1C VWD, there is a normal propeptide level even when the antigen is low, because the mature VW protein was created after cleavage and may have been cleared out of circulation as a downstream process. In type 3 VWD, however, because of inability to produce any VWF, both the antigen and propeptide levels are low [7].

Management Options

The management and follow-up of type 3 VWD are similar to hemophilia, as significant and spontaneous bleeding complications can be seen. Desmopressin does not lead to an adequate increase in VWF or FVIII levels in type 3 disease and hence, is not a viable therapeutic option.

Factor replacement constitutes the mainstay of therapy. Both plasma-derived and recombinant VWF concentrates are commercially available for replacement, but FDA approval for recombinant products in children is pending in the United States (Table 11.1). These products are typically marketed with the information of their VWF (in RCo units) and FVIII contents and can be selected based on the highest VWF/FVIII ratio. Most of the VWF concentrate products have VWF:RCo/FVIII ratio over 1, providing more VWF than FVIII, but both these levels should be monitored after infusion. The FVIII levels may go higher than as

Table 11.1 Available plasma-derived and recombinant von Willebrand concentrates

Product name	Manufacturer	Type of product	Processing of product	VWF:RCo/ FVIII content (ratio ± SD)
Humate P®	CSL Behring	Monoclonally derived, plasma-based	Produced after multiple precipitation procedures, pasteurization or sterilization	1.6–2.7
Alphanate®	Grifols	Plasma-derived	Heparin ligand chromatography, dry heat viral inactivation	0.5
Koate-DVI®[a]	Grifols/ Kedrion/BD Pharma	Plasma-derived	gel permeation chromatography, heat inactivation	0.8–1.2
Wilate®[a]	Octapharma	Plasma-derived	Ion exchange + size exclusion chromatography	0.9
Vonvendi®	Baxalta	Recombinant	Purified rVWF from Chinese hamster ovary has trace of mouse as well	No factor VIII

[a]Not available in the United States/not FDA approved for VWD

expected with the concentrate alone, because the endogenous FVIII produced in these patients now survives after VWF infusion. Some centers choose to dose and monitor therapy based on FVIII levels after ensuring initial increase in VWF levels.

> Factor VIII concentrates that are monoclonally purified or recombinant do not contain sufficient VWF to be able to use them in VWD. In the absence of VWF, FVIII alone will not survive in circulation to effect adequate hemostasis.

The recombinant von Willebrand factor (rVWF) concentrate that is FDA approved for clinical use in adults requires specific modification to dosing compared to plasma-derived VWF concentrates. Because this product contains no FVIII, if it is being utilized in a pre-surgical setting, the first dose should be administered at least 6–8 hours before the procedure, such that the VWF can stabilize endogenous FVIII in the patient. The subsequent doses can be given as any other VWF product, as the endogenous FVIII will be chaperoned and survive in the circulation. In the setting of acute bleeding, however, without endogenous FVIII, rVWF is not suitable for adequate hemostasis, unless accompanied by a FVIII concentrate, at least for the first dose. Similar target levels and doses for FVIII, as in hemophilia patients, can be utilized for such a single dose. For VWF, the target troughs per Table 11.2 should be utilized for rVWF as well. The advantage of using rVWF is that when multiple successive doses of VWF replacement are required, it does not lead to significantly high levels of FVIII [8].

General goals of replacement therapy are to maintain adequate VWF levels based on the type of injury during a bleeding event and the time until healing and hemostasis can occur. Thus, factor dosages, frequency, and duration for need for therapy vary for different clinical scenarios. Table 11.2 provides a general guideline that can be utilized in various scenarios based on past literature [4, 9, 10].

Cryoprecipitate contains VWF, along with FVIII, factor XIII, and fibrinogen, and was previously used for replacement therapy. With availability of virally inactivated and more concentrated replacement factor proteins, the use of cryoprecipitate is discouraged in VWD. In resource-limited settings, without a clear diagnosis, and in the absence of the VWF concentrates, cryoprecipitate can be used to control bleeding. One must weigh its benefits against the risk, as it does carry a risk of infection transmission. Each cryoprecipitate donor unit (i.e., one bag) contains approximately 100 units of VWF and FVIII. Fresh frozen plasma or FFP is an even more nonspecific and less concentrated form of VWF replacement. It should be considered as a last resort therapy in undiagnosed bleeding disorder patients,

Table 11.2 VWF concentrate dosing based on different indications in severe VWD

Type of procedure/ bleed risk	Goal trough level for VWF:RCo	Dose based on VWF:RCo			Therapy guidance
		Loading dose (IU/Kg)	Maintenance dose[a] (IU/Kg)	Infusion frequency	
Minor surgery or small procedures	>30–50%	40–50 (or 20–40)	If needed, can be 40–50 (1–2 doses may be sufficient)	Every 8–12 hours needed to complete 2–5 days of hemostasis	Therapy can be supported with antifibrinolytics if in areas of high fibrinolysis
Major surgery	>80–100% for first 2–4 days, then >50% until good healing	40–60	40–60 IU	Every 8–12 hours needed for 2–4 days then daily	Total duration of therapy can be 7–14 days based on expected healing and, after about 7–10 days of levels ~50%, can taper to bring to ~30% for the next 3–5 days to ensure healing and no secondary hemorrhage
Dental extraction	>50%	30–40	Not needed unless bleeding is seen		Antifibrinolytics for 5–7 days
Menorrhagia	>50%	40–50	40–50	Single daily dose	Antifibrinolytics for 5 days per month
Delivery and postpartum period	>100% initially, then >50%	40–60	40–50	12–24 hours	Antifibrinolytics for 7–14 days

| Other clinically significant bleeding[b] | >50–80% or >100% initially (based on location and risk) | 40–60 | 40–50 | Every 8–12 hours needed until hemostasis then daily | Therapy can be supported with antifibrinolytics if in areas of high fibrinolysis |

IU international units, *kg* kilograms, *VWF:RCo* von Willebrand factor levels based on ristocetin cofactor units

[a]For example, tongue/oropharynx hematoma, eye- or other organ-threatening bleeding, joint bleeding

[b]Need for frequent maintenance infusions should be based on invasiveness of procedure and pharmacokinetic measures and recovery in each patient

as it has a small amount of all factors. Each unit provides about 1% improvement in circulating levels of VWF, and a significant risk of volume overload accompanies its use in replacement therapy.

Nonfactor Therapies

DDAVP-based therapies are not effective in raising VWF levels in patients with type 3 VWD due to inadequate VWF stores in the Weibel-Palade bodies. Antifibrinolytic agents are commonly utilized as adjunctive therapies in patients with VWD.

Anticipatory Guidance

All precautions that are advised for patients with hemophilia apply to type 3 and severe VWD patients. Patients with type 3 VWD should be cautioned against use of nonsteroidal anti-inflammatory drugs (NSAIDs) and anticoagulants due to increased bleeding risk. Patients should be encouraged to use protective gear and sporting guards; and avoid high-impact and high-velocity activities. Regular dental cleaning is advised to maintain tooth and gum health and avoid oral bleeds. All invasive procedures should be planned with the advice of the hematology team.

Antibodies to VWF

About 5–10% of patients with type 3 VWD may develop alloantibodies after being exposed to replacement factor [11]. Patients with homozygous gene deletions or nonsense mutation-related etiologies are more likely to develop alloantibodies. These patients typically will not respond to VWF replacement. They may additionally be at risk for life-threatening anaphylaxis in response to VWF infusion. For emergent or major bleeding episodes, alternative therapy with recombinant coasulation factor VIIa (FVIIa) is a therapeutic option.

Prophylaxis in VWD

Patients with type 3 VWD with frequent and spontaneous bleeding episodes can benefit from regular prophylaxis and close surveillance to monitor for complications. As these patients can also be prone to joint damage and life-threatening bleeding events, regular replacement therapy may prove very useful in preventing long-term morbidity [12]. The common indications for starting prophylaxis include frequent/severe nose and mouth bleeding, joint bleeding, and/or gastrointestinal (GI) bleeding (in relation to angiodysplasia) [13]. Findings from the prophylaxis studies suggest substantial reduction in annualized bleeding rates, improvement in frequency of debilitating GI and oropharyngeal bleeding, as well as reduced incidence of arthropathy in patients that start young (<5 years of age) [14]. Dosing for prophylaxis can vary and is based on the clinical picture and vascular access, but the most commonly used regimens, utilizing around 50 IU/dL of VWF:RCo, are given once to three times a week.

Outcomes and Follow-Up

Among the types of VWD, type 3 disease is associated with high morbidity and poor prognosis without appropriate therapy. Hemophilia treatment centers (HTCs) have hematologists and other physicians experienced in caring for the unique issues seen in type 3 VWD, along with access to products and appropriate therapeutic agents and appropriate laboratory testing.

With appropriate management and regular follow-up in specialized hematology centers, the life-threatening and debilitating aspects of type 3 disease can be addressed.

> A discussion about regular/biannual follow-up at an HTC and about initiating regular prophylaxis (especially if there are frequent spontaneous bleeding events) in our index case study patient should also be considered.

Clinical Pearls and Pitfalls
- DDAVP is not effective in patients with type 3 VWD.
- Differentiation of type 3 VWD from severe type 1 VWD, type 1C disease, and hemophilia A should be made based on family history, personal history, and laboratory evaluation.
- Regular prophylaxis is effective at preventing debilitating joint bleeds and other severe bleeding events.
- Inhibitory antibodies occur in 5–10% of patients with type 3 VWD.
- Recombinant VWF does not contain FVIII; thus, initial treatment of active bleeds requires an additional source of FVIII.

References

1. Labarque V, Stain AM, Blanchette V, Kahr WH, Carcao MD. Intracranial haemorrhage in von Willebrand disease: a report on six cases. Haemophilia. 2013;19(4):602–6.
2. Flood VH, Gill JC, Friedman KD, Bellissimo DB, Haberichter SL, Montgomery RR. Von Willebrand disease in the United States: a perspective from Wisconsin. Semin Thromb Hemost. 2011;37(5):528–34.
3. Lillicrap D. Genotype/phenotype association in von Willebrand disease: is the glass half full or empty? J Thromb Haemost. 2009;7(Suppl 1):65–70.
4. Nichols WL, Hultin MB, James AH. Von Willebrand disease (VWD): evidence- based diagnosis and management guidelines, the National Heart, Lung, and Blood Institute (NHLBI) Expert Panel report (USA). Haemophilia. 2008;14:171–232.
5. Castaman G, Rodeghiero F, Tosetto A, Cappelletti A, Baudo F, Eikenboom JC, et al. Hemorrhagic symptoms and bleeding risk in obligatory carriers of type 3 von Willebrand disease: an international, multicenter study. J Thromb Haemost. 2006;4(10):2164–9.
6. Montgomery RR. When it comes to von Willebrand disease, does 1 + 1 = 3? J Thromb Haemost. 2006;4(10):2162–3.
7. Haberichter SL. von Willebrand factor propeptide: biology and clinical utility. Blood. 2015;126(15):1753–61.

8. Rodeghiero F, Castaman G, Tosetto A. How I treat von Willebrand disease. Blood. 2009;114(6):1158–65.
9. Mannucci PM. Treatment of von Willebrand's disease. N Engl J Med. 2004;351(7):683–94.
10. Leebeek FWG, Eikenboom JCJ. Von Willebrand's disease. N Engl J Med. 2016;375(21):2067–80.
11. James PD, Lillicrap D, Mannucci PM. Alloantibodies in von Willebrand disease. Blood. 2013;122(5):636–40.
12. Berntorp E. Prophylaxis in von Willebrand disease. Haemophilia. 2008;14(Suppl 5):47–53.
13. Abshire T, Cox-Gill J, Kempton CL, Leebeek FW, Carcao M, Kouides P, et al. Prophylaxis escalation in severe von Willebrand disease: a prospective study from the von Willebrand Disease Prophylaxis Network. J Thromb Haemost. 2015;13(9):1585–9.
14. Saccullo G, Makris M. Prophylaxis in von Willebrand disease: coming of age? Semin Thromb Hemost. 2016;42(5):498–506.

Pathophysiology and Management of Acquired von Willebrand Syndrome

12

Dominder Kaur and Sarah H. O'Brien

Case Presentation You are consulted on an 8-year-old male with history of Ebstein's anomaly, aberrant right subclavian artery, and initial tricuspid valve replacement complicated by venoarterial extracorporeal membranous oxygenation (VA-ECMO) postoperatively, who recently underwent Glenn procedure and right ventricular plication, followed by tricuspid valve replacement 1 week later. Recent procedure was also complicated

---

D. Kaur (✉)
Department of Pediatrics, Division of Pediatric Hematology/Oncology/Stem Cell Transplant, Columbia University Irving Medical Center, Children's Hospital of New York/New York Presbyterian Morgan Stanley Children's Hospital, New York, NY, USA
e-mail: dk3076@cumc.columbia.edu

S. H. O'Brien
Nationwide Children's Hospital, Division of Pediatric Hematology, Oncology and Bone Marrow Transplant, Columbus, OH, USA

Center for Innovation in Pediatric Practice, Abigail Wexner Research Institute at Nationwide Children's Hospital, Columbus, OH, USA

Department of Pediatrics, The Ohio State University College of Medicine, Columbus, OH, USA
e-mail: Sarah.Obrien@nationwidechildrens.org

by the need for VA-ECMO, and he had hemodynamic instability related to bleeding post chest tube closure, responsive to volume resuscitation. He was stable for the subsequent day with his hemodynamic status improving and labs stabilizing. You are now consulted because yesterday evening, he developed bleeding from chest wound, from his nares, and around chest tubes, requiring heparin to be held. Cardiology and the intensive care units are concerned about acquired von Willebrand disease, as he had similar issues when he was on ECMO the last time.

Multiple Choice Management Question

You will send off which among the following evaluations?

(a) Coagulation screen with prothrombin time (PT) and activated partial thromboplastin time (aPTT)
(b) Platelet function analysis (PFA)
(c) Von Willebrand antigen and activity levels
(d) Multimer distribution evaluation
(e) **All of the above**

> This is a patient context wherein acquired von Willebrand disease is high on the differential. The initial evaluation can begin with a complete blood count (CBC), prothrombin time (PT), activated partial thromboplastin time (aPTT), PFA, von Willebrand panel (antigen and activity levels), factor VIII level, and VW multimer evaluation. Hence, the answer is e.

Epidemiology, Clinical Presentation, and Pathophysiology

Acquired von Willebrand syndrome (AVWS), as the name suggests, occurs due to acquired defects of the von Willebrand factor – and can be qualitative or quantitative. It is a rare bleeding disorder that can develop in susceptible populations and requires a high index of suspicion for correct diagnosis.

Due to the possibility of being underreported and underdiagnosed, its true incidence remains unclear, but estimates from 0.04% to 5% occurrence in the susceptible populations have been reported [1].

As evidenced by the case example above, AVWS often occurs in the setting of a complicated medical background. Concurrent anticoagulation therapy and quantitative or qualitative platelet issues may be present simultaneously and make initial evaluation difficult.

AVWS is common in patients with congenital cardiac diseases or postsurgical anatomical cardiac configurations. The most commonly implicated lesion is aortic stenosis. Patients who are on left or other ventricular assist devices (VAD) or extracorporeal membrane oxygenation (ECMO) additionally are at high risk of developing AVWS. Such AVWS often has a rapid onset and can occur within a week of initiating such mechanical support [2]. In children, Wilms tumor is known to be associated with AVWS. Patients on certain medications, along with those with glycogen storage diseases and autoimmune conditions like systemic lupus erythematosus (SLE) or hypothyroidism, may also present with this defect.

The underlying hemostatic defect emanates from loss of high, and sometimes intermediate, molecular weight von Willebrand multimers. With the most active areas of the protein being lost, the interactions between the von Willebrand factor (VWF) protein, subendothelium, and platelets are adversely affected. Additionally, a low circulatory factor VIII (FVIII) level may result due to reduced protection from its carrier protein. All of these issues together lead to an increased bleeding risk, which may manifest as mucocutaneous bleeding or deeper organ/tissue bleeding due to low FVIII.

There are multiple postulated mechanisms for acquired VWD. These can be broadly categorized as immune-related or otherwise. Nonimmune mechanisms can affect both production and proteolysis of the VWF. Decreased production leading to AVWS is seen in hypothyroidism and possibly in patients on valproic acid therapy [3]. Other drugs implicated in AVWS include few antimicrobials (e.g., ciprofloxacin, griseofulvin) and hydroxyethyl starch [4].

Increased proteolysis in the setting of high-shear flow rate environments, is the primary mechanism in populations with underlying cardiac pathologies and circulatory support devices, e.g., aortic stenosis, ventricular septal defects, and VADs/ECMO (Fig. 12.1). In these high-shear high-flow-rate vascular environments, the globular conformation of VWF is unfurled into a linear form, and this exposes the A2 domain. With this change, the cryptic ADAMTS13 binding sites become open and available, resulting in proteolytic loss of the high molecular weight (HMW) multimers. Heyde syndrome is the classic example of such acquired type 2 VWD in patients with aortic stenosis, which manifests with angiodysplasia and gastrointestinal bleeding [5]. Modified flow dynamic in pulmonary hypertension also leads to similar proteolysis.

The pathophysiology in myeloproliferative disorders and thrombocytotic scenarios is different – with cellular adsorption of VWF being the underlying mechanism. Increased binding of the hemostatic HMW multimers occurs onto the more numerous cells in essential thrombocythemia, reactive thrombocytosis, polycythemia vera, or some other tumor cells [6]. This results in effective removal of these complexes from circulation. Partial reduction in available VWF, due to some of it remaining platelet bound, also contributes to the acquired VWF deficiency [7].

Immune-related mechanisms include antibody-mediated clearance or inhibition of VWF. Cell-mediated or drug-induced clearance of VWF also fall in the immune category. These autoimmune mechanisms can also be seen in the lymphoproliferative diseases and malignancies and have also been implicated in SLE.

Differential Diagnosis

The differential for AVWS includes other acquired bleeding disorders and platelet dysfunction. As AVWS often occurs in complex medical situations, other etiologies for bleeding like synthetic or consumptive coagulopathies (e.g., liver failure or disseminated intravascular coagulation/DIC) and acquired conditions, like thrombotic thrombocytopenic purpura or atypical hemolytic

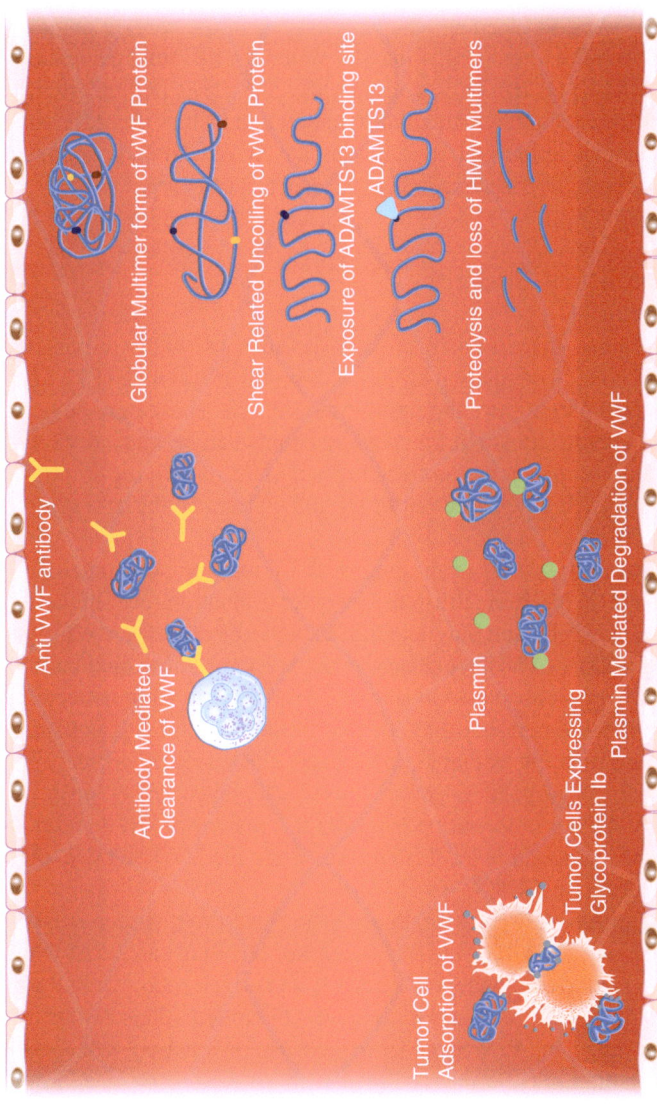

Fig. 12.1 Pathophysiology and mechanisms leading to development of acquired von Willebrand disease

uremic syndrome, should be considered. Overanticoagulation with supratherapeutic heparin or warfarin levels or platelet inhibition leading to bleeding, can also happen in the cardiac population. Acquired hemophilia may be similar in its initial evaluation as FVIII levels can be low in both these diseases but underlying mechanism and the patient presentation and history are different. It becomes important to differentiate AVWS from congenital VWD because the management approaches can vary.

Laboratory Findings

Laboratory evaluation in AVWS should start with a complete blood count, coagulation screen with prothrombin time (PT), and activated partial thromboplastin time (aPTT). These may be normal in some cases, but low platelet counts can be seen, if VWF-platelet complexes are produced as part of the underlying etiology, as these will be cleared out of the circulation. In the absence of other platelet inhibition/dysfunction, a PFA can also prove quite sensitive to AVWS. A prolonged aPTT may be seen when the FVIII level has been affected. The other evaluations are similar to those in VWD, and may identify decreased values for VWF:Ag, VWF:RCo, or FVIII. A change in the VWF multimer distribution can be very informative in showing a decrease in large molecular weight multimers but may also be normal at times. If collagen binding assay is available, it will also show similar decrease in binding. If propeptide testing is available, an increased propeptide/VWF:Ag ratio will be seen. Being a marker of VWF production, the propeptide level is normal, while the VWF antigen will be reduced in AVWS.

Multimer distribution pattern is the closest to that seen in type 2A among the VWD variants. At times, bleeding can occur with only a reduction in the VWF activity to antigen ratio, while their absolute values remain within acceptable ranges. This can be an early stage in AVWS; and on multimer evaluation, abnormal distribution may be seen, helping with the diagnosis. New onset of mucocutaneous bleeding in an at-risk patient population should stimulate consideration for AVWS. Personal history of previously normal hemostasis and a negative family history, also prove useful in differentiating acquired from congenital VWD. Genetic testing to confirm this may not always be available in a timely manner.

In immune-mediated pathologies, like lymphoproliferative disorders, detection of VWF antibodies may aid AVWS diagnosis. Caution should be exercised while utilizing this testing for diagnosis, as a low rate of antibody detection is reported. This could be due to assay limitations, as well as due to poor detection of some of the antibodies because of them remaining bound to the VWF. Non-neutralizing antibodies are easier to detect and can be identified on enzyme-linked immunosorbent assays (ELISA) [8]. VWF survival testing after VWF infusion or DDAVP administration, may prove useful in some settings [4].

Management

The management goals in AVWS are to stop and prevent bleeding events, as well as to take steps toward reversal or remission of the disease-causing defect. An important aspect of AVWS management is taking prophylactic measures when high-risk situations are identified.

Desmopressin or DDAVP (at a dose of 0.3 µg/kg per dose, with maximum 20 µg) is useful for acute bleeding events in AVWS as for a short term; it leads to new VWF being released from endothelial cells. A DDAVP response evaluation is recommended and should be carried out whenever feasible. This can help differentiate complete and partial responders and nonresponders. DDAVP is most effective for immune-mediated AVWS, but some improvement can also be seen in cardiovascular or thrombocytosis pictures, wherein proteolysis and adsorptive mechanisms of disease are in play. Due to its ability to transiently increase VWF, DDAVP can be used as prophylaxis for minor hemostatic challenges in other patients as well, once they are identified to be responders (e.g., patient with aortic stenosis or thrombocytosis). When using DDAVP, one must remain mindful of its effects on fluid balance and possibility of hyponatremia.

Von Willebrand factor concentrates are useful in AVWS as well. They may be needed in patients wherein a sustained response cannot be obtained with DDAVP alone or when there is significant bleeding despite DDAVP and additional support is needed, before a dose can be repeated for concern of tachyphylaxis. VWF concentrates are dosed based on the ristocetin cofactor units, or on the factor FVIII units in the product. An initial dose can be 50 to 100 RCo IU/kg, and further dosing is based on the response. With both DDAVP and VWF replacement therapies, pharmacokinetic studies with post-dose levels prove helpful in guiding frequency of therapy and future doses. Such recovery levels are especially useful in the setting of neutralizing VWF antibodies.

Antifibrinolytics are a useful adjunctive therapy for AVWS, especially when DDAVP or VWF replacement is being utilized. The commonly used forms are epsilon aminocaproic acid and tranexamic acid, which are both lysine analogs that work via inhibition of plasmin activity on fibrin. They may suffice alone for minor bleeding events in areas with high fibrinolytic activity, like the mouth or the gut. They are also helpful for menstrual bleeding and small oral/dental procedures.

Use of recombinant factor VIIa (rFVIIa) is indicated in patients with anti-VWF alloantibodies and severe bleeding. The basis of its use is similar to hemophilia therapy in the setting of an inhibitor and rFVIIa works as a bypassing agent. Thus, dosing similar to that used in hemophilia, i.e., 90 µg/kg, can be utilized. The data on this are relatively limited, and there is associated thrombosis risk, that one should remain cautious of [9].

> For our case, DDAVP and VWF factor concentrate can be considered as therapies. If DDAVP is successful in stopping bleeding, antifibrinolytic therapy can also be used as an adjunct, while being mindful of the thrombosis risk. In the absence of bleeding, supportive care is sufficient. If there is bleeding and it is too early to repeat DDAVP, VWF concentrate can be given. Plans for coming off ECMO should be frequently discussed, as permitted by the hemodynamic stability. Once ECMO is removed, AVWS reverses rather quickly.

Additional adjunctive efforts to minimize bleeding, like maintaining safe platelet counts in the complicated patients with systemic and multiorgan issues and optimizing anticoagulation to avoid bleeding, are important management components.

Underlying mechanical, malignant, and autoimmune conditions leading to AVWS also make this condition just as amenable to reversal. With surgical correction, chemotherapy, or immunosuppression, AVWS also improves. For significant immunological diseases like lupus, systemic therapy with intravenous immunoglobulins or plasmapheresis or agents like steroids or cyclophosphamide may be indicated [10]. Whenever underlying issues can be addressed, steps toward such therapies should be considered an integral part of AVWS management.

Outcomes and Follow-Up

Most of the patients that develop AVWS due to a treatable condition, can revert to normal VWF levels. For patient with Wilms tumor or thrombocythemic issues, chemotherapy-related remission can also normalize VWF levels. For underlying cardiac issues, once corrective surgery is performed and the shearing anatomy is gone, VWF defects also improve. Normalization of the multimer pattern and improvement in the VWF:Ag/RCo ratio confirm reversal of the defect. For patients that are on circulatory support devices like VAD or ECMO, AVWS is promptly and completely reversed after device is explanted. The immune-mediated AVWS may be more difficult to treat and be persistent, but can improve with effective immunosuppression.

Due to etiologies in AVWS being heterogeneous, there is need for individualizing care. Most patients have a positive outcome with regard to disease reversal after correction of the underlying issue and, thus, have a good prognosis. Follow-up frequency can be based on the disease activity and bleeding risk.

In the absence of bleeding issues, follow-up can be annually for patients with persistent AVWS. Once steps toward correction for the underlying issue are taken, one immediate follow-up and another a few months out, with repeat VWF panel at the latter, should be planned. By 1 year from correction, almost all patients show reversal of the AVWS. Being a complex and heterogeneous disease, patients with AVWS should be cared for by hematologists with expertise in this disease or at a hemophilia treatment center (HTC).

> **Clinical Pearls and Pitfalls**
> - A high level of suspicion in the correct clinical setting and appropriate timing of laboratory evaluation are essential to establish the correct diagnosis of acquired VWD in a timely manner.
> - Anticoagulant and platelet inhibition therapy can make correct diagnosis difficult in patients with underlying complex cardiac conditions and in those who are on vascular support devices.
> - Although multimer testing is helpful in identifying AVWS, for acute bleeding in sick patients, there may not always be sufficient time to wait for multimer distribution results. It is prudent to then make the diagnosis based on patient's personal and family history, new onset of VWF defects, and decreased VWF:RCo to VWF:Ag ratio.
> - For patients who develop AVWS while on mechanical support with VAD and ECMO, the VWF profile defects and related bleeding risk normalize soon after they come off such devices.
> - DDAVP/desmopressin may be successfully used for small procedures in AVWS.
> - Angiodysplasia and related GI bleeding can also be seen in patients with AVWS, and this phenomenon in Heyde syndrome has contributed to identification of role of VWF in angiogenesis. Once the underlying cardiac defect is corrected, the angiodysplasia also improves.

References

1. Franchini M, Lippi G. Acquired von Willebrand syndrome: an update. Am J Hematol. 2007;82(5):368–75.
2. Heilmann C, Geisen U, Beyersdorf F, Nakamura L, Benk C, Berchtold-Herz M, et al. Acquired von Willebrand syndrome in patients with ventricular assist device or total artificial heart. Thromb Haemost. 2010;103(5):962–7.
3. Callaghan MU, Wong TE, Federici AB. Treatment of acquired von Willebrand syndrome in childhood. Blood. 2013;122(12):2019–22.
4. Nichols WL, Hultin MB, James AH. Von Willebrand disease (VWD): evidence- based diagnosis and management guidelines, the National Heart, Lung, and Blood Institute (NHLBI) Expert Panel report (USA). Haemophilia. 2008;14:171–232.
5. Loscalzo J. From clinical observation to mechanism–Heyde's syndrome. N Engl J Med. 2012;367(20):1954–6.
6. Veyradier A, Jenkins CS, Fressinaud E, Meyer D. Acquired von Willebrand syndrome: from pathophysiology to management. Thromb Haemost. 2000;84(2):175–82.
7. Budde U, van Genderen PJ. Acquired von Willebrand disease in patients with high platelet counts. Semin Thromb Hemost. 1997;23(5):425–31.
8. Tiede A. Diagnosis and treatment of acquired von Willebrand syndrome. Thromb Res. 2012;130(Suppl 2):S2–6.
9. Tiede A, Rand JH, Budde U, Ganser A, Federici AB. How I treat the acquired von Willebrand syndrome. Blood. 2011;117(25):6777–85.
10. Kumar R, Steele M. Acquired bleeding disorders in children. In: Blanchette VSBV, Revel-Vilk S, editors. SickKids handbook of pediatric thrombosis and hemostasis, vol. 1. 2nd ed. Basel: Karger; 2017. p. 134–56.

Part IV

Thrombocytopenias

Approach to a Patient with Sudden Onset of Mucocutaneous Bleeding and Thrombocytopenia

Melissa J. Rose and
Amanda Jacobson-Kelly

Case Presentation A 2-year-old previously healthy male presents with 3-day history of recurrent epistaxis, easy bruising, and petechial rash. Each bleeding episode from his nose lasts less than 5 minutes but has been happening at least twice a day. He and the rest of his family had an upper respiratory infection 2–3 weeks ago. They deny bleeding from his gums, hematuria, or blood in his stool. He has not had fevers, weight loss, bone or joint complaints, night sweats, or "lumps/bumps." There is no family history of bleeding disorders, autoimmune disease, early hearing loss, or kidney disease. On physical examination, he is active and well-

M. J. Rose (✉) · A. Jacobson-Kelly
Nationwide Children's Hospital, Division of Pediatric Hematology, Oncology and Bone Marrow Transplant, Columbus, OH, USA

Department of Pediatrics, The Ohio State University College of Medicine, Columbus, OH, USA
e-mail: Melissa.Rose@NationwideChildrens.org;
Amanda.Jacobson@NationwideChildrens.org

© Springer Nature Switzerland AG 2020
A. L. Dunn et al. (eds.), *Pediatric Bleeding Disorders*,
https://doi.org/10.1007/978-3-030-31661-7_13

appearing with scattered bruises on his forehead, trunk, and extremities. His left nare is obstructed with dried blood. There are no oral lesions, lymphadenopathy, hepatosplenomegaly, or skeletal deformities. CBC and the peripheral blood smear are normal aside from a platelet count of 18,000/mm^3 and a few large platelets seen.

Differential Diagnosis

As acute ITP is a diagnosis of exclusion, other categories of etiologies must be considered:

- *Inherited bleeding disorders* such as *MYH9*-related disorders (associated with hearing defects and renal disease), Bernard-Soulier syndrome, congenital amegakaryocytic thrombocytopenia (CAMT), type 2B von Willebrand disease, thrombocytopenia-absent radius (TAR), X-linked thrombocytopenia, and familial platelet disorder with predisposition to MDS/AML (RUNX1). Most of these are likely to have had previous bleeding history and often have more severe bleeding symptoms.
- *Acquired bone marrow suppression/failure* such as postinfectious, toxic exposure, medication side effect, and aplastic anemia.
- *Bone marrow replacement*, as in leukemia or metastatic disease.
- *Increased platelet consumption* in the setting of some infections, sepsis, and thrombotic microangiopathy.
- Finally, the clinical picture, without thrombocytopenia, can be concerning for *child abuse*.

Multiple Choice Management Question

The diagnosis of ITP requires:

A. Analysis of a bone marrow aspirate and biopsy with cytogenetic assessment
B. **Thorough history, physical exam, and review of peripheral blood smear**
C. Detection of platelet autoantibodies

Diagnosis and Nomenclature

The International Working Group consensus panel, composed of adult and pediatric experts, provides definitions and terminology as below:

Primary immune thrombocytopenia is defined as a platelet count less than 100,000/mm^3 without another cause. *Secondary ITP* can be associated with antiphospholipid antibody syndrome, Evans syndrome, common variable immune deficiency, drug administration, infections (such as Epstein-Barr virus, cytomegalovirus, *Helicobacter pylori*, hepatitis C, HIV, varicella) lymphoproliferative disorders, vaccination, or lupus [1, 2].

Acute ITP has been subcategorized into *newly diagnosed*, from diagnosis to 3 months, and *persistent*, 3–12 months from diagnosis. Patients with immune thrombocytopenia for more than 12 months are considered to have *chronic ITP* [1, 2].

When a thorough history, physical examination, and review of the CBC and peripheral blood smear are consistent with ITP, no further testing is required for the diagnosis of ITP. Specifically, bone marrow examination is not necessary for diagnosis or prior to medical management. Evaluation for platelet autoantibodies has also not proven to be of benefit, as their presence does not eliminate other etiologies of thrombocytopenia and their absence does not negate the clinical ITP diagnosis. Low-level autoantibodies may be missed, and only limited select platelet glycoproteins are used.

Patients clinically present with mucocutaneous bleeding symptoms, such as epistaxis, gingival bleeding, ecchymoses, purpura and/or hematomas, petechiae, hematuria, blood in the stool, or increased menstrual bleeding. "Red flag" symptoms or exam findings, such as unexplained or persistent fever, weight loss, night sweats, bony or joint pain, severe headaches, enlarged lymph nodes or hepatosplenomegaly, and abnormal thumbs or forearms, should prompt further evaluation for an etiology other than ITP. Additionally, acute ITP is less likely with an insidious onset. Underlying inherited thrombocytopenias or autoimmune disease, respectively, should be more strongly considered in patients presenting less than 1 year of age or greater than 10 years of age. Personal or family history of renal disease and/or sensorineural hearing loss should prompt consideration for *MYH9*-related disorders.

Most patients can be managed in the outpatient setting, aside from those with serious bleeding. The definition of severe bleeding is not standardized, making reporting and ability to compare among completed studies difficult. Examples of serious bleeding include epistaxis lasting >5–15 minutes, gastrointestinal bleeding, or other mucosal bleeding that results in anemia that could, or does, require transfusion and intracranial hemorrhage (ICH). Severe, non-ICH bleeding has been reported in approximately 3% of children; ICH has been reported in 0.2–0.6% of pediatric patients with ITP and more likely in patients with chronic rather than acute ITP [3, 4].

Epidemiology

The incidence of ITP is approximately 1.9–6.4 per 100,000 children per year, with most patients presenting between 2 and 5 years of age [5]. In children less than 1 year, there is a slight male predominance with the male/female ratio of 1.7:1, yet the opposite is true for adolescents and young adults, where there is a slightly higher female predominance. This leaves an overall male/female ratio of 1.2:1 throughout childhood [6]. There is seasonal variation in presentation, although no specific identifiable cause.

Pathophysiology

The predominant etiology for ITP is increased platelet clearance. This is due to aberrant generation of platelet autoantibodies and heightened phagocytosis of these antibody-platelet complexes by the spleen. Additionally, in some cases, autoantibodies directed against megakaryocytes are responsible for impaired megakaryocyte maturation, as well as apoptosis and phagocytosis [7].

Laboratory Findings

A complete blood count will demonstrate a platelet count <100,000/mm^3, with otherwise normal white blood cell count and differential, no anemia, and normal red blood cell morphology. The size of the platelets is generally large, but not giant (Fig. 13.1).

The immature platelet fraction represents platelets that are early in their lifespan and can be distinguished by their increased RNA content, detectable via flow cytometry; this is generally elevated in patients with acute ITP [8, 9].

Management

In 1996, the American Society of Hematology published a comprehensive guideline for the diagnosis and treatment of ITP. This was updated in 2011, in regard to definitions and treatment, and again in 2019, primarily for management.

The goal of management of ITP in children is not to attain a normal platelet count, but to achieve adequate hemostasis, with strong emphasis on health-related quality of life (HRQoL). For children with no or mild bleeding, observation for worsening bleeding symptoms and expectant management is recommended,

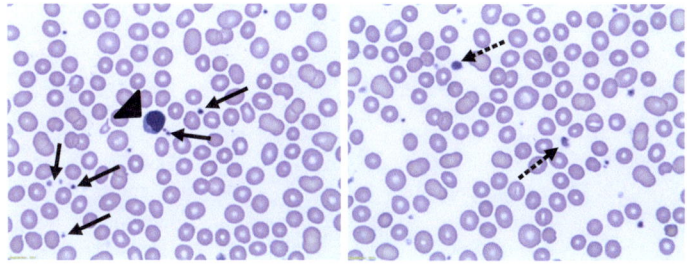

Fig. 13.1 Peripheral blood smear (PBS) of ITP. A normal PBS on the left with a typical lymphocyte (arrowhead), normal red cell morphology, and normal distribution of platelets (arrows) all being approximately the same size. An ITP PBS on the right demonstrating variety in platelet size with a population of larger platelets (dash arrows)

regardless of the platelet count, given the very low risk of intracranial hemorrhage or life-threatening bleeding. A discussion with the family should include assessment for appropriate access to care, level of bleeding risk due to activity level or behavior concerns, and any need for surgical procedures; after anticipatory guidance on monitoring for bleeding and education on the profiles of potential medical management options, a mutual decision can be reached [2–4].

First-line therapies include corticosteroids, intravenous immunoglobulin (IVIg), and anti-D immunoglobulin (Table 13.1). The development of severe hemorrhage was not found to be related to initial management; thereby, no one treatment has been shown to clearly benefit patients, short term or long term [3]. Corticosteroids are relatively inexpensive and an attractive oral outpatient therapy. They impair antibody-antigen clearance and decrease antibody production. Short-term side effects with "steroid burst" mostly include moodiness, behavior changes, increased appetite, sleep difficulties, and possibly gastritis, with other side effects such as hyperglycemia and hypertension predominantly occurring with more long-term therapy regimens. One potential but exceedingly

Table 13.1 Options for first-line management of ITP

	Dose	Time to response	Side effects
Observation and education	Time	1–3 weeks	Anxiety (parental) Bleeding
Corticosteroids	Prednisone: 4 mg/kg PO divided BID for 4 days (usual max 60–80 mg BID) Dexamethasone: 40 mg once daily for 4 days	Initial 2–14 days Peak 4–28 days	Irritability Gastritis Hypertension Hyperglycemia Delay leukemia diagnosis
IVIg	0.8–1.0 gm/kg IV for one dose	Initial 1–3 days Peak 2–7 days	Infusion reaction Headache Aseptic meningitis
Anti-D Immunoglobulin	75 mcg/kg IV for one dose	Initial 1–3 days Peak 3–7 days	Hemolysis FDA black box warning

rare risk with steroids is the misdiagnosis of ITP for leukemia and, thus, partial treatment with steroid initiation. Meeting all of the diagnosis parameters for ITP is of utmost importance, and if there is concern for malignancy, then alternative therapies should be initiated. IVIg incurs higher medical costs related to the medication itself, as well as administration needs, as this is a several-hour infusion. IVIg reduces phagocytic clearance of platelets via transient receptor blockade and decreases secretion and increases clearance of the autoantibodies. IVIg has a faster initial platelet response than steroids. Headache and vomiting are common side effects and may be symptoms of aseptic meningitis. Infusion of anti-D immunoglobulin induces immunoglobulin-coated red blood cells, which compete with the platelet-autoantibody complexes for reticuloendothelial clearance. The infusion is shorter than IVIg, and cost is slightly less. It cannot be used in those who are Rh negative, and a decline in hemoglobin of approximately 2 g is expected, so it should not be administered to patients with anemia or concerns for autoimmune hemolysis. There is an FDA black box warning for life-threatening hemolysis with specific recommendations for clinical and laboratory monitoring post infusion.

Patients may be retreated with these medications, or second-line therapies, such as thrombopoietin (TPO) receptor agonists, rituximab, splenectomy, and nonsteroidal immunosuppressive medications, could be considered (see chapter on chronic ITP).

Little evidence-based guidance exists to support or refute recommendations for restrictions or limitations on activities in patients with ITP. Using the American Academy of Pediatrics Council on Sports Medicine and Fitness' classification of contact, limited contact, or noncontact sports, one survey of approximately 60 subjects was queried on level of participation, with subgroup analysis based on platelet counts. While approximately one-fourth of subjects reported injuries across 10 different sports, higher incidences of injury were associated with higher contact levels but not with lower platelet counts. The authors concluded that sports participation is likely too restricted and children with ITP should be encouraged to be athletic [10]. A survey of pediatric hematologist/oncologists revealed significant variation in physician perception of contact risk for different sports. Differing medical advice on sport restrictions for patients with ITP was expressed, with many physicians recommending against "moderate risk" sports participation when platelet counts were <50,000/mm^3 and against any sports participation when platelet counts were <25,000/mm^3; authors expressed concerns that this could negatively impact HRQoL and encouraged family-physician shared decision-making for individualized participation recommendations [11].

Future Considerations

Investigation into identifying possible genetic predisposition to ITP is currently underway. Additionally, the search for biomarkers that could indicate duration of disease or response to therapy is ongoing. Eltrombopag, a TPO receptor agonist approved for pediatric chronic ITP, is being studied for initial and duration of platelet response, as well as time to resolution of disease, in subjects with acute ITP.

Clinical Pearls and Pitfalls
- Acute immune thrombocytopenia (ITP) is the most common acquired bleeding disorder with peak presentation in the preschool age group, characterized by sudden onset of mucocutaneous bleeding.
- Diagnosis is that of exclusion and can be made with a thorough history, physical exam, CBC only showing a platelet count <100,000/mm^3, and blood smear with few large platelets; bone marrow assessment is not necessary for diagnosis.
- Pay due attention to "red flags" at presentation, including personal history and age at presentation, family history, physical exam, laboratory findings, etc., to avoid misdiagnosis and partial treatment of leukemia with corticosteroids.
- The thrombocytopenia culminates from autoantibody production, increased platelet removal, and, at times, reduced platelet production.
- Typical management may include careful observation, corticosteroids, IVIg, and/or anti-D immunoglobulin.

References

1. Rodeghiero F, Stasi R, Gernsheimer T, Michel M, Provan D, Arnold DM, Bussel JB, Cines DB, Chong BH, Cooper N, Godeau B, Lechner K, Mazzucconi MG, Mcmillan R, Sanz MA, Imbach P, Blanchette V, Kühne T, Ruggeri M, George JN. Standardization of terminology, definitions and outcome criteria in immune thrombocytopenic purpura of adults and children: report from an international working group. Blood. 2009;113(11):2386–93.
2. Neunert C, Lim W, Crowther M, Cohen A, Solberg L Jr, Crowther MA, American Society of Hematology. The American Society of Hematology 2011 evidence-based practice guideline for immune thrombocytopenia. Blood. 2011;117(16):4190–207.
3. Neunert CE, Buchanan GR, Imbach P, Bolton-Maggs PH, Bennett CM, Neufeld EJ, Vesely SK, Adix L, Blanchette VS, Kühne T, Intercontinental Childhood ITP Study Group Registry II Participants. Severe hemorrhage in children with newly diagnosed immune thrombocytopenic purpura. Blood. 2008;112(10):4003.
4. Neunert C, Noroozi N, Norman G, Buchanan GR, Goy J, Nazi I, Kelton JG, Arnold DM. Severe bleeding events in adults and children with primary immune thrombocytopenia: a systematic review. J Thromb Haemost. 2015;13(3):457.
5. Terrell DR, Beebe LA, Vesely SK, Neas BR, Segal JB, George JN. The incidence of immune thrombocytopenic purpura in children and adults: a critical review of published reports. Am J Hematol. 2010;85(3):174–80.
6. Kühne T, Imbach P, Bolton-Maggs PH, Berchtold W, Blanchette V, Buchanan GR, Intercontinental Childhood ITP Study Group. Newly diagnosed idiopathic thrombocytopenic purpura in childhood: an observational study. Lancet. 2001;358(9299):2122–5.
7. Wei A, Jackson SP. Boosting platelet production. Nat Med. 2008;14(9):917–8.
8. Barsam SJ, Psaila B, Forestier M, Page LK, Sloane PA, Geyer JT, Villarica GO, Ruisi MM, Gernsheimer TB, Beer JH, Bussel JB. Platelet production and platelet destruction: assessing mechanisms of treatment effect in immune thrombocytopenia. Blood. 2011;117(21):5723–32.
9. Adly AA, Ragab IA, Ismail EA, Farahat MM. Evaluation of the immature platelet fraction in the diagnosis and prognosis of childhood immune thrombocytopenia. Platelets. 2015;26(7):645.
10. Brigstocke S, McGuinn CE, Bussel JB. Sports participation in children with ITP: a case for liberalization? Blood. 2012;120:Abstract 3339.
11. Kumar M, Lambert MP, Breakey V, Buchanan GR, Neier M, Neufeld EJ, Kempert P, Neunert CE, Nottage K, Klaassen RJ, ITP Consortium of North America. Sports participation in children and adolescents with Immune Thrombocytopenia (ITP). Pediatr Blood Cancer. 2015;62:2223–5.

A Preteen Female with Fatigue and Incidental Finding of Thrombocytopenia

14

Melissa J. Rose and
Amanda Jacobson-Kelly

Case Presentation A 12-year-old female presented 1 year ago to her primary care provider with complaints of fatigue, with an otherwise negative history. A complete blood count (CBC) was obtained and notable for a normal white blood cell count and hemoglobin, as well as red blood cell indices, yet the platelet count was low at 32,000/mm^3. The primary care provider reviewed her history, and she had a CBC at 2 years of age with a platelet count of 253,000/mm^3. This physician has been monitoring the patient clinically and with serial CBC. She has had mild bruising with injuries but no other bleeding concerns, and the platelet count has ranged from 22 to 85,000/mm^3, most recently 78,000/mm^3. The primary physician referred the patient to you, the hematologist, as the thrombocytopenia has not resolved and the patient is in need of molar teeth extraction. The patient and family denied a history of infections or need for antibiotics. Non-bleeding review of symptoms includes lack of visual or hearing concerns, oral ulcerations or lesions, chest pain or shortness of breath, abdominal pain or abnormal bowel habits, hematuria, rashes, and joint pain or swelling. She has not yet begun menstruating. There is a family history in second-degree relatives for a variety of autoimmune diseases, including Hashimoto's thyroiditis, psoriasis, and lupus. The spleen tip is just palpable below the left costal margin with deep palpation, and there are quarter- and nickel-sized bruises on her left and right shin, respectively; physical examination is otherwise normal. Review of the peripheral blood smear demonstrated reduced platelet numbers with few large platelets, normal white blood cell differential, and red cell morphology.

Multiple Choice Management Question

What *supportive* care therapy could be prescribed for this patient's upcoming dental surgery?

A. Aspirin/NSAID
B. **Antifibrinolytic agent**
C. Thrombopoietin receptor agonist (TPO-RA)

While there are no completed randomized control trials to assess efficacy of antifibrinolytic agents in patients with ITP, case reports and expert opinions report of their usefulness in patients with thrombocytopenia for prevention of recurrent bleeding or bleeding with minor surgical procedures [1]. Aspirin and NSAIDs impair platelet function and should be avoided, to minimize compounded bleeding risk. TPO-RAs are generally considered therapeutic and not supportive therapy. Additionally, primary endpoints for clinical trials involving these agents have been a platelet count $\geq 50{,}000/\text{mm}^3$ and reduction in bleeding risk. In this patient without bleeding symptoms and platelet count $>50{,}000/\text{mm}^3$, as well as surgical procedure unlikely to result in significant bleeding, antifibrinolytic agents as needed would be the best answer for supportive therapy.

Differential Diagnosis

The differential diagnosis of chronic ITP includes that of acute ITP, as noted in the previous chapter. *Inherited thrombocytopenia disorders*, such as *MYH9*-related disorders, Bernard-Soulier syndrome, and familial platelet disorder with predisposition to MDS/AML (*RUNX1*) often having more severe bleeding symptoms, would not have demonstrated a normal platelet count in the past, and many will have additional indicative family history. *Bone marrow failure or bone marrow replacement*, as with myelodysplastic syndrome, is another possible diagnosis for chronic thrombocytopenia. Additionally, ITP itself could be secondary to *autoimmune diseases* (antiphospholipid antibody syndrome, Evans syndrome, lupus), *immunodeficiency* or *immune dysregulatory states* (lymphoproliferative disorders such as autoimmune lymphoproliferative syndrome (ALPS), common variable immunodeficiency), or *chronic infections* (HIV, hepatitis C, *Helicobacter pylori*).

Epidemiology and Pathophysiology

The estimated prevalence of chronic ITP is 4.6/100,000 children [2, 3]. As discussed in a previous chapter, a majority of pediatric patients with ITP will have resolution of thrombocytopenia, with the rate of remission in children of 69% by 6 months. For those with chronic ITP, remission rate between 12 and 24 months from diagnosis is 28% [4, 5]. Female patients, those who receive the diagnosis after 10 years of age, and those with presenting platelet counts above 20,000/mm^3 are more likely to have the diagnosis of chronic ITP [3, 6]. While additional clinical or laboratory biomarkers have attempted to predict the development of chronic versus acute ITP, none of these have been consistent across studies.

As with acute ITP, the pathophysiology for chronic ITP is directly related to increased platelet clearance, but additionally, ineffective thrombopoiesis plays a prime role in chronic ITP [7]. Chronic secondary ITP may be attributed to chronic infections or immune dysregulatory/autoimmune disorders, yet this remains rare. Therefore, the initial American Society of Hematology guidelines, as well as the update in 2011, did not recommend routine testing in children for antiplatelet antibodies, antiphospholipid antibodies, or infectious etiologies, such as HIV, hepatitis C, or *Helicobacter pylori*, unless they are otherwise clinically indicated [4, 8].

Non-hematologic Manifestation

As illustrated in the case, fatigue is often reported in adult and pediatric patients with chronic ITP, with approximately 8% of children missing work or school, not due to bleeding symptoms, but because of fatigue [9]. In a prospective, multicenter observational study, fatigue was self-reported in 36% of children and 37% of adolescents with ITP. This was not significantly different from that reported by children and adolescents with cancer (34% and 21%, respectively), using the same fatigue scale [10]. Practitioners should recognize the relevance of this non-hematologic symptom when considering treatment. Further investigation into the association between fatigue and thrombocytopenia is needed.

Management Options

First-Line Therapies

The Intercontinental Cooperative ITP Study Group reported on their cohort of 1345 subjects that cutaneous bleeding is the most common bleeding symptom in patients with chronic ITP; there were no events of intracranial hemorrhage in their registry that spanned 2001–2007. As major hemorrhage was rare, despite prolonged thrombocytopenia in many patients, therapy is generally recommended for those with bleeding symptoms [11]. First-line therapies, such as IVIG, anti-D immunoglobulin, and corticosteroids, as previously described for acute ITP, may be used in the same intermittent manner for patients with chronic ITP.

Second-Line Therapies

Immunomodulatory agents, including mycophenolate, sirolimus, rituximab, dapsone, danazol, azathioprine, cyclophosphamide, vinca alkaloids, and cyclosporine, have been used in patients with chronic ITP with variable outcomes. The time to response tends to be days to months for most of these agents, and toxicities are medication specific. While collective response rates approximate 70%, there have not been randomized control trials to show superior efficacy of any of these medications in pediatric patients with ITP [1]. That being said, some of these immunomodulatory agents have shown benefit in select patient populations with secondary ITP. For example, mycophenolate and sirolimus are recommended for treatment of immune cytopenias associated with ALPS [12, 13].

Rituximab is a chimeric monoclonal antibody directed against CD20, a surface marker on B lymphocytes, which are responsible for producing antibodies. Typical dosing is 375 mg/m^2 weekly for 4 weeks, yet other dosing regimens such as 100 mg/m^2 weekly for 4 weeks or 1 gram (adult flat dose) every other week for two total doses have shown similar overall and complete responses [14, 15]. The most common side effects are infusion reactions and serum sickness in pediatric patients. Viral reactivation of hepatitis B is possible, so patients should be screened prior to administration [1]. Overall response rates after rituximab are about 60% in refractory ITP, yet pediatric patients have decreased long-term response compared to adults, as sustained responses were only seen in 33% of children at 1 year and 26% at 5 years [16]. Infectious complications are rare in ITP patients, despite the inability to produce antibody for a period of time. There is minimal decline in overall immunoglobulin by the time there is repopulation of B lymphocytes, which commonly occurs between 6 and 12 months after administration. On the other hand, in some patients with ALPS, CVID, Evans syndrome, or other immunodeficiency syndromes, persistent hypogammaglobulinemia, impaired antibody responses, and prolonged neutropenia have been reported after rituximab [4, 12].

There are currently two TPO-RA agents, eltrombopag and romiplostim, that are FDA approved for use in pediatric patients with chronic ITP. Both have reported response rates of approximately 80% and minimal long-term toxicity or significant adverse events [4]. Eltrombopag is a once daily oral medication (with dietary restriction related to interaction with divalent cations such as calcium and iron) that gained approval for treatment of chronic ITP in children in 2015. Tablets should not be crushed, but a liquid formulation has been prepared and intermittently available. Eltrombopag undergoes hepatic metabolism, so monitoring for hepatotoxicity is recommended; hepatotoxicity is reversible, should it occur. Animal studies raised concern for cataract development, but this has not been clearly demonstrated in the adult or pediatric trials, yet monitoring is recommended [17, 18]. Romiplostim is a once-weekly subcutaneous injection that was approved for pediatric patients in 2018. Ease of dose modifications and lack of dietary restrictions are tempered with injection site discomfort. There was an initial concern for reversible bone marrow fibrosis in the adult studies, but this was not found in the pediatric studies; bone marrow assessment is only recommended if concerns are raised on review of the peripheral blood smear or response to therapy declines. Inability for home administration remains a deterrent for some [18]. While some patients have been able to wean and discontinue these therapies, the majority of patients remain on these medications long term.

Splenectomy offers remission rates estimated to be 54% in children with ITP, yet splenectomy has been recommended less in the last several years [4, 5, 19]. This is multifactorial. First, despite vaccination and prophylactic antimicrobials, the risk of postsplenectomy sepsis remains as high as 3% in children [1]. This risk for infection-related morbidity and mortality is especially true in patients with ALPS. Secondly, such patients with secondary ITP due to ALPS, Evans syndrome, or other disorders of immune regulation may also be less likely to respond to splenectomy [20–22]. Additionally, maintenance medical options, such as TPO-RAs, are well-tolerated, effective, and more readily available with FDA approval. Finally, there is an increased incidence of thrombosis following splenectomy, compounding the potential long-term complications of this procedure.

Little evidence and no randomized controlled trials exist to guide recommendations in the choice of second-line therapies. To begin to address this issue, the ITP Consortium of North America performed a prospective, multicenter observational study of 120 children starting second-line treatments, specifically rituximab, other oral immunosuppressive agents, TPO-RAs, and splenectomy, which examined treatment decisions and therapeutic responses. Treating physicians rated patient/parental preference and treatment factors (side effect profile, long-term toxicity, ease of administration, possibility of remission, and perceived efficacy) as top reasons for selecting therapies [23]. All treatments increased platelet counts and demonstrated improvements in health-related quality of life (HRQoL) scores, with romiplostim having the greatest effect on platelet counts at 6 months and patients treated with eltrombopag having achieved a minimal important difference at 1 month in the HRQoL assessment tool [24]. Comparative effectiveness studies are needed to further guide shared decision-making.

Outcomes and Follow-Up

There are no guidelines for frequency of serial laboratory testing or assessments for this chronic disease, and most practitioners encourage patients to obtain labs with clinical symptoms and with clinical visits at least semiannually. Patients receiving medical therapy should follow monitoring parameters specific to that therapy. Practitioners should have a high index of suspicion for etiologies of secondary ITP, with laboratory testing based on clinical concerns.

Clinical Pearls and Pitfalls
- Chronic ITP is rare in pediatric patients but can have a significant impact on HRQoL, with hematologic and non-hematologic symptoms, particularly fatigue.
- One should remain vigilant and assess for underlying etiologies for chronic thrombocytopenia, such as inherited thrombocytopenia disorders, as well as evaluation of secondary causes of ITP, for example, immune dysregulation disorders, immunodeficiencies, chronic infections, or autoimmune diseases.
- Several maintenance treatment options are available, yet no randomized control trials or comparative studies are available to demonstrate superiority or provide guidelines for care. Shared informed decision-making between practitioners and patient/parents is recommended.

References

1. Provan D, Stasi R, Newland AC, Blanchette VS, Bolton-Maggs P, Bussel JB, Chong BH, Cines DB, Gernsheimer TG, Godeau B, Grainger J, Greer I, Hunt BJ, Imbach PA, Lyons G, McMillan R, Rodeghiero F, Sanz MA, Tarantino M, Watson S, Young J, Kuter DJ. International consensus report on the investigation and management of primary immune thrombocytopenia. Blood. 2010;115(2):168–860.
2. Fogarty PF, Segal JB. The epidemiology of immune thrombocytopenic purpura. Curr Opin Hematol. 2007;14:515–9.
3. Del Vecchio GC, De Santis A, Accettura L, De Mattia D, Giordano P. Chronic immune thrombocytopenia in childhood. Blood Coagul Fibrinolysis. 2014;25(4):297–9.
4. Despotovic JM, Grimes AB. Pediatric ITP: is it different from adult ITP? Hematology Am Soc Hematol Educ Program. 2018;2018(1):405–11.
5. Schifferli A, Holbro A, Chitlur M, et al. Intercontinental Cooperative ITP Study Group (ICIS). A comparative prospective observational study of children and adults with immune thrombocytopenia: 2-year follow-up. Am J Hematol. 2018;93(6):751–759.
6. Glanz J, France E, Xu S, Hayes T, Hambidge S. A population-based, multisite cohort study of the predictors of chronic idiopathic thrombocytopenic purpura in children. Pediatrics. 2008;121:e506–12.

7. Wei A, Jackson SP. Boosting platelet production. Nat Med. 2008; 14(9):917–8.
8. Neunert C, Lim W, Crowther M, Cohen A, Solberg L Jr, Crowther MA, American Society of Hematology. The American Society of Hematology 2011 evidence-based practice guideline for immune thrombocytopenia. Blood. 2011;117(16):4190–207.
9. Sarpatwari A, Watson S, Erqou S, et al. Health-related lifestyle in adults and children with primary immune thrombocytopenia (ITP). Br J Haematol. 2010;151(2):189–91.
10. Grace R, Despotovic J, Bennett C, et al. Fatigue in pediatric immune thrombocytopenia (ITP): baseline prevalence in patients starting second line therapies in the first ITP Consortium of North America research study (ICON1). Pediatr Blood Cancer. 2016;63:S20.
11. Neunert CE, Buchanan GR, Imbach P, Bolton-Maggs PHB, Bennett CM, Neufeld E, Vesely SK, Adix L, Blanchette VS, Kühne T for the Intercontinental Cooperative ITP Study Group Registry II Participants. Bleeding manifestations and management of children with persistent and chronic immune thrombocytopenia: data from the Intercontinental Cooperative ITP Study Group (ICIS). Blood. 2013;121:4457–62.
12. Rao VK, Oliveira JB. How I treat autoimmune lymphoproliferative syndrome. Blood. 2011;118(22):5741–51.
13. Teachey D. New advances in the diagnosis and treatment of autoimmune lymphoproliferative syndrome. Curr Opin Pediatr. 2012;24:1–8.
14. Li Y, Shi Y, He Z, Chen Q, Liu Z, Yu L, Wang C. The efficacy and safety of low-dose rituximab in immune thrombocytopenia: a systematic review and meta-analysis. Platelets. 2019;30(6):690–7.
15. Khellaf M, Charles-Nelson A, Fain O, Terriou L, Viallard JF, Cheze S, Graveleau J, Slama B, Audia S, Ebbo M, Le Guenno G, Cliquennois M, Salles G, Bonmati C, Teillet F, Galicier L, Hot A, Lambotte O, Lefrère F, Sacko S, Kengue DK, Bierling P, Roudot-Thoraval F, Michel M, Godeau B. Safety and efficacy of rituximab in adult immune thrombocytopenia: results from a prospective registry including 248 patients. Blood. 2014;124(22):3228–36.
16. Patel VL, Mahevas M, Lee SY, et al. Outcomes 5 years after response to ´rituximab therapy in children and adults with immune thrombocytopenia. Blood. 2012;119(25):5989–95.
17. Kim TO, Despotovic J, Lambert MP. Eltrombopag for use in children with immune thrombocytopenia. Blood Adv. 2018;2:454–61.
18. Neunert CE, Rose MJ. Romiplostim for the management of pediatric immune thrombocytopenia: drug development and current practice. Blood Adv. 2019;3(12):1907–15.
19. Bhatt NS, Bhatt P, Donda K, et al. Temporal trends of splenectomy in pediatric hospitalizations with immune thrombocytopenia. Pediatr Blood Cancer. 2018;65(7):e27072.

20. Price S, Shaw PA, Seitz A, et al. Natural history of autoimmune lymphoproliferative syndrome associated with FAS gene mutations. Blood. 2014;123(13):1989–99.
21. Teachey DT, Manno CS, Axsom KM, et al. Unmasking Evans syndrome: T-cell phenotype and apoptotic response reveal autoimmune lymphoproliferative syndrome (ALPS). Blood. 2005;105(6):2443–8.
22. Seif AE, Manno CS, Sheen C, Grupp SA, Teachey DT. Identifying autoimmune lymphoproliferative syndrome in children with Evans syndrome: a multi-institutional study. Blood. 2010;115(11):2142–5.
23. Grace RF, Despotovic JM, Bennett CM, Bussel JB, Neier M, Neunert C, Crary SE, Pastore YD, Klaassen RJ, Rothman JA, Hege K, Breakey VR, Rose MJ, Shimano KA, Buchanan GR, Geddis A, Haley KM, Lorenzana A, Thompson A, Jeng M, Neufeld EJ, Brown T, Forbes PW, Lambert MP. Physician decision making in selection of second-line treatments in immune thrombocytopenia in children. Am J Hematol. 2018;93(7):882–8.
24. Grace RF, Shimano KA, Bhat R, Neunert C, Bussel JB, Klaassen RJ, Lambert MP, Rothman JA, Breakey VR, Hege K, Bennett CM, Rose MJ, Haley KM, Buchanan GR, Geddis A, Lorenzana A, Jeng M, Pastore YD, Crary SE, Neier M, Neufeld EJ, Neu N, Forbes PW, Despotovic JM. Second-line treatments in children with immune thrombocytopenia: effect on platelet count and patient-centered outcomes. Am J Hematol. 2019;94(7):741–50.

Diagnosis and Management of an Infant with Microthrombocytopenia

15

Melissa J. Rose and
Amanda Jacobson-Kelly

Case Presentation You are referred a 6-month-old male infant to your hematology clinic for evaluation of petechiae. The infant also has significant eczema and has been evaluated by dermatology who prescribed topical steroids for treatment. His mother reports that his eczema symptoms have only slightly improved despite good adherence to use of topical steroids and routine eczema care. She reports first noticing intermittent petechiae several months ago, typically located on his trunk and extremities. Occasionally, she will see petechiae on his face, where he

---

M. J. Rose (✉) · A. Jacobson-Kelly
Nationwide Children's Hospital, Division of Pediatric Hematology, Oncology and Bone Marrow Transplant, Columbus, OH, USA

Department of Pediatrics, The Ohio State University College of Medicine, Columbus, OH, USA
e-mail: Melissa.Rose@NationwideChildrens.org;
Amanda.Jacobson@NationwideChildrens.org

© Springer Nature Switzerland AG 2020
A. L. Dunn et al. (eds.), *Pediatric Bleeding Disorders*,
https://doi.org/10.1007/978-3-030-31661-7_15

scratches eczematous lesions. Petechiae seem more numerous recently. Additionally, his mother reports that he bruises easily, even noting bruising on his back from picking him up, which she finds unusual. She denies other bleeding symptoms.

He is a product of a full-term, uncomplicated pregnancy. Eczema began around 3 months of life. He has had two episodes of pneumonia, one that required hospitalization for 4 days with IV antibiotics. He has also had four ear infections since 4 months of age.

On exam, he is a well-developed, well-nourished infant. Vital signs and weight are normal for age. His skin exam is significant for scattered eczematous plaques on his cheeks, scalp, trunk, and extremities. He has scattered petechiae on his trunk and extremities as well as a few on his scalp (shown in Fig. 15.1). The remainder of his exam is normal.

Complete blood count (CBC) reveals thrombocytopenia (platelet count 50,000/microL). Hemoglobin and white blood cell count are normal. Peripheral blood smear reveals small platelets that are reduced in number.

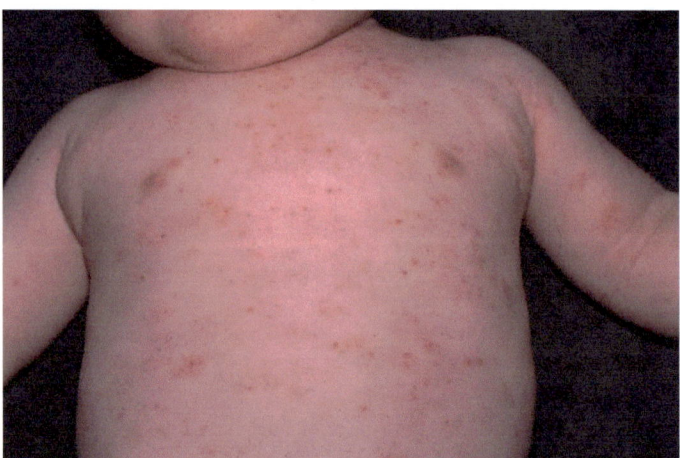

Fig. 15.1 This photo demonstrates eczematous lesions and scattered petechiae on the infant's trunk. The presence of petechiae in addition to eczema is more specific for WAS. Typical infants with eczema will not have petechiae

Multiple-Choice Management Question

In addition to a CBC and peripheral smear, what additional testing would be MOST helpful in identifying the disease causing this infant's symptoms?

(a) Platelet function analysis
(b) **WAS protein (WASp) by flow cytometry**
(c) Platelet aggregation studies

Differential Diagnosis

The differential diagnosis for this infant includes inherited and acquired thrombocytopenias. The duration of symptoms (petechiae ongoing for several months), young age, and overall non-ill appearance of the infant go against an acute or acquired cause making an inherited thrombocytopenia most likely. The size of the patient's platelets provides another clue in diagnosis. Inherited thrombocytopenias with a normal platelet size include thrombocytopenia absent radii (TAR) syndrome, amegakaryocytic thrombocytopenia with radioulnar synostosis (ARTUS), as well as other bone marrow failure syndromes including congenital amegakaryocytic thrombocytopenia (CAMT), Fanconi anemia, dyskeratosis congenita, and Shwachman-Diamond syndrome. The differential diagnosis for an inherited thrombocytopenia with a small platelet size (inherited microthrombocytopenia) is less broad and includes Wiskott-Aldrich syndrome (WAS) and X-linked thrombocytopenia (XLT). This patient has small platelets, so one of these is most likely.

In this clinical case, the diagnosis is classic WAS. WAS is characterized by a triad of (1) severe immune dysregulation resulting in recurrent infections, autoimmune disease, and lymphoid malignancies, (2) thrombocytopenia with small platelets, and (3) eczema. Eczema is secondary to immune dysregulation. The bleeding phenotype in patients with classic WAS is varied. WAS has X-linked inheritance and thus should be considered in any male patient with unexplained thrombocytopenia and autoimmunity or frequent infections [1].

Management Options

Management options for patients with classic WAS are supportive initially. Hematopoietic stem cell transplant (HSCT) is the only available curative option. Gene therapy, as an alternative to HSCT, is currently under investigation. These will be discussed in more detail below.

Supportive Management

Platelet transfusion should be used to treat major bleeding episodes and/or prior to surgery. Otherwise, routine platelet transfusion for bleeding prevention is not recommended due to the risk of alloimmunization. Blood products should be irradiated and tested for cytomegalovirus given immunodeficiency in these patients. Eltrombopag, an oral thrombopoietin receptor agonist that has been approved to treat thrombocytopenia in children with immune thrombocytopenia, may be useful to increase platelet count in patients with WAS and to avoid need for platelet transfusion prior to HSCT [2].

Prophylactic trimethoprim-sulfamethoxazole, dapsone, or pentamidine should be given to prevent *P. jirovecii* pneumonia in young patients with classic WAS. Intravenous immunoglobulin therapy (IVIg) should be given to any WAS patient with antibody deficiency [3]. Due to the immune dysregulation and particularly autoimmune cytopenias present in these patients, immunosuppressive therapy may be required prior to transplant. Rituximab, a monoclonal antibody targeting the B-cell CD20 antigen, has been shown to be safe and effective in classic WAS patients already receiving IVIg. It is essential for these patients to receive IVIg in conjunction with rituximab to ameliorate the increased risk of infection due to inability to mount an antibody response subsequent to rituximab therapy [4]. Splenectomy was previously utilized as a treatment option in patients with WAS to increase circulating platelet counts, especially in patients without a suitable donor for HSCT [5]. This treatment is falling out of favor, as more options for HSCT donors become available including haploidentical donor transplants [6]. All WAS patients who undergo splenectomy should be on lifelong antibiotic prophylaxis to prevent infection with encapsulated organisms.

Curative Options

Among the inherited thrombocytopenias, HSCT is rarely utilized as a treatment option with the exception of classic WAS [1]. Human leukocyte antigen (HLA)-matched sibling donor HSCT is the ideal option with the best outcome (approximately 90% 5-year survival), with HSCT outcomes continuing to improve in the last two decades [7, 8]. Currently, survival following matched unrelated donor HSCT is approaching that of patients who receive matched sibling donor transplants. The outcome of mismatched and haploidentical donor HSCT is improving but remains substantially lower than HSCT with a matched donor [9, 10]. HSCT is most successful if performed when the patient is <5 years of age at the time of transplant [8, 9, 11]. Myeloablative regimens are recommended over reduced intensity regimens due to the risk of graft rejection [12].

Gene therapy, in which a normal *WAS* gene copy is introduced into hematopoietic stem cells isolated from a WAS patient and then manipulated cells are given back to the patient following a reduced intensity conditioning regimen, is a potentially curative therapy for WAS that is currently being studied [13, 14].

Laboratory Findings

On CBC, the only initial finding may be thrombocytopenia with a low mean platelet volume (MPV). Platelet counts generally range between 20,000 and 50,000/microL. Peripheral smear will show

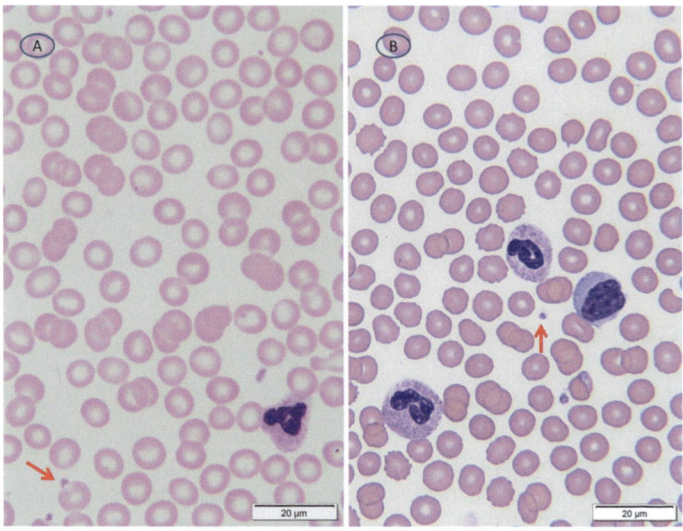

Fig. 15.2 Microthrombocytes seen in WAS. Panel A shows a normal peripheral blood smear. Panel B shows a peripheral blood smear with microthrombocytes (red arrows) from a patient with WAS. (The image is provided by Samir B. Kahwash, MD. Department of Pathology and Laboratory Medicine, Nationwide Children's Hospital, Columbus, OH)

microthrombocytopenia (Fig. 15.2). Though immunodeficiency is present, total white blood cell count may be unaffected. Absolute lymphocyte count may be decreased but is often normal in infancy [15]. Examination of serum immunoglobulins may show low IgG and IgM and often elevated IgA and IgE. Patients will often have inadequate antibody responses to vaccines. B- and T-cell immunophenotype may show a decreased number of T lymphocytes.

Flow cytometry can be used to screen for the presence or absence of the WAS protein (WASp) using an anti-WASp antibody; however, this testing may miss patients with dysfunctional WASp [16]. The clinical phenotype of WAS can correlate with the presence or absence of WASp expression. Genetic sequencing for *WAS* gene mutations is required for proper diagnosis [17]. Mutations in the *WAS* gene result in classic WAS or a less severe form called X-linked thrombocytopenia (XLT) and X-linked neutropenia (XLN), which will be discussed below.

Epidemiology and Inheritance/Genetics

Epidemiology

WAS is rare with an incidence of approximately 1 in 100,000 live births. It is an X-linked disease and thus occurs almost exclusively in males. About 50% of patients with the *WAS* gene mutation have a classic WAS phenotype, and the remainder have a XLT phenotype. XLN is very rare and has only been reported in less than a dozen patients [18].

Inheritance/Genetics

The *WAS* gene is located on the short arm of the X chromosome. Mutations in the *WAS* gene have three distinct phenotypes based on the type of mutation and the degree of WASp expression. Classic WAS is the most severe form, typically resulting from deletions, insertions, and nonsense mutations in the *WAS* gene and absent WASp expression [17, 19].

Patients with XLT have a less severe variant, most commonly a result of missense mutations, leaving some WASp production [19]. XLT is characterized by the presence of thrombocytopenia with small platelets yet without the immune deficiency that occurs in classic WAS. Eczema may be present but is typically very mild. Patients with XLT do have an increased risk of malignancies, but the risk is lower than in patients with classic WAS [20]. There is a much rarer entity described in two families known as intermittent X-linked thrombocytopenia with small platelet size in which a missense mutation in the *WAS* gene was found. These patients did not have other clinical features of WAS and had adequate WASp expression [21].

XLN, also a result of *WAS* gene mutations, is a rare form of severe congenital neutropenia characterized by increased infections related to neutropenia, as well as lymphocyte dysfunction. These patients are also at increased risk for myelodysplastic syndrome [22].

Outcomes and Follow-Up

Patients with classic WAS have substantially reduced life expectancies due to death from infections, bleeding, autoimmune disease, or malignancy. Therefore, HSCT at an early age, if a suitable donor is available, is paramount in their management. Gene therapy is a potentially promising option for patients without a suitable donor. Patients with XLT typically have life expectancies similar to that of an unaffected male [18].

Patients with severe WAS are followed routinely by hematology and immunology, until HSCT, at which time care is often transitioned to the transplant team.

> **Clinical Pearls and Pitfalls**
> - The differential diagnosis for an inherited thrombocytopenia with a small platelet size (inherited microthrombocytopenia) includes WAS and XLT.
> - WAS is characterized by a triad of (1) severe immune dysregulation resulting in recurrent infections, autoimmune disease, and lymphoid malignancies, (2) thrombocytopenia with small platelets, and (3) eczema.
> - WAS has X-linked inheritance and thus should be considered in any male patient with early-onset thrombocytopenia with small platelet size or unexplained thrombocytopenia with autoimmunity or frequent infections.
> - Management options for patients with classic WAS are supportive initially with prophylactic antimicrobials, prompt initiation of antibiotics for infections, antifibrinolytic agents for mild bleeding, and irradiated platelet transfusions reserved for significant bleeding symptoms or prior to surgeries.
> - Hematopoietic stem cell transplant (HSCT) is the only available curative option. Gene therapy is an alternative to HSCT that is currently under investigation.

- Flow cytometry to screen for the presence or absence of WASp may be useful, but genetic testing is required to confirm the diagnosis.
- XLT is a less severe form of WAS. Patients with XLT typically have some WASp expression and lack the immune deficiency present in WAS.
- XLN and X-linked intermittent thrombocytopenia are very rare entities resulting from mutations in the *WAS* gene

References

1. Balduini CL, Iolascon A, Savoia A. Inherited thrombocytopenias: from genes to therapy. Haematologica. 2002;87(8):860–80.
2. Gerrits AJ, Leven EA, Frelinger AL 3rd, et al. Effects of eltrombopag on platelet count and platelet activation in Wiskott-Aldrich syndrome/X-linked thrombocytopenia. Blood. 2015;126(11):1367–78.
3. Blaese RM, Strober W, Levy AL, Waldmann TA. Hypercatabolism of IgG, IgA, IgM, and albumin in the Wiskott-Aldrich syndrome. A unique disorder of serum protein metabolism. J Clin Invest. 1971;50(11):2331–8.
4. Kim JJ, Thrasher AJ, Jones AM, Davies EG, Cale CM. Rituximab for the treatment of autoimmune cytopenias in children with immune deficiency. Br J Haematol. 2007;138(1):94–6.
5. Mullen CA, Anderson KD, Blaese RM. Splenectomy and/or bone marrow transplantation in the management of the Wiskott-Aldrich syndrome: long-term follow-up of 62 cases. Blood. 1993;82(10):2961–6.
6. Kharya G, Nademi Z, Leahy TR, et al. Haploidentical T-cell alpha beta receptor and CD19-depleted stem cell transplant for Wiskott-Aldrich syndrome. J Allergy Clin Immunol. 2014;134(5):1199–201.
7. Shin CR, Kim MO, Li D, et al. Outcomes following hematopoietic cell transplantation for Wiskott-Aldrich syndrome. Bone Marrow Transplant. 2012;47(11):1428–35.
8. Filipovich AH, Stone JV, Tomany SC, et al. Impact of donor type on outcome of bone marrow transplantation for Wiskott-Aldrich syndrome: collaborative study of the International Bone Marrow Transplant Registry and the National Marrow Donor Program. Blood. 2001;97(6):1598–603.
9. Moratto D, Giliani S, Bonfim C, et al. Long-term outcome and lineage-specific chimerism in 194 patients with Wiskott-Aldrich syndrome

treated by hematopoietic cell transplantation in the period 1980-2009: an international collaborative study. Blood. 2011;118(6):1675–84.
10. Friedrich W, Schutz C, Schulz A, Benninghoff U, Honig M. Results and long-term outcome in 39 patients with Wiskott-Aldrich syndrome transplanted from HLA-matched and -mismatched donors. Immunol Res. 2009;44(1–3):18–24.
11. Kobayashi R, Ariga T, Nonoyama S, et al. Outcome in patients with Wiskott-Aldrich syndrome following stem cell transplantation: an analysis of 57 patients in Japan. Br J Haematol. 2006;135(3):362–6.
12. Ozsahin H, Cavazzana-Calvo M, Notarangelo LD, et al. Long-term outcome following hematopoietic stem-cell transplantation in Wiskott-Aldrich syndrome: collaborative study of the European Society for Immunodeficiencies and European Group for Blood and Marrow Transplantation. Blood. 2008;111(1):439–45.
13. Aiuti A, Biasco L, Scaramuzza S, et al. Lentiviral hematopoietic stem cell gene therapy in patients with Wiskott-Aldrich syndrome. Science. 2013;341(6148):1233151.
14. Morris EC, Fox T, Chakraverty R, et al. Gene therapy for Wiskott-Aldrich syndrome in a severely affected adult. Blood. 2017;130(11):1327–35.
15. Ochs HD, Slichter SJ, Harker LA, Von Behrens WE, Clark RA, Wedgwood RJ. The Wiskott-Aldrich syndrome: studies of lymphocytes, granulocytes, and platelets. Blood. 1980;55(2):243–52.
16. Chiang SCC, Vergamini SM, Husami A, et al. Screening for Wiskott-Aldrich syndrome by flow cytometry. J Allergy Clin Immunol. 2018;142(1):333–335 e338.
17. Imai K, Morio T, Zhu Y, et al. Clinical course of patients with WASP gene mutations. Blood. 2004;103(2):456–64.
18. Wiskott-Aldrich syndrome. 2018. www.uptodate.com. Accessed 26 June 2019.
19. Jin Y, Mazza C, Christie JR, et al. Mutations of the Wiskott-Aldrich Syndrome Protein (WASP): hotspots, effect on transcription, and translation and phenotype/genotype correlation. Blood. 2004;104(13):4010–9.
20. Albert MH, Bittner TC, Nonoyama S, et al. X-linked thrombocytopenia (XLT) due to WAS mutations: clinical characteristics, long-term outcome, and treatment options. Blood. 2010;115(16):3231–8.
21. Notarangelo LD, Mazza C, Giliani S, et al. Missense mutations of the WASP gene cause intermittent X-linked thrombocytopenia. Blood. 2002;99(6):2268–9.
22. Ancliff PJ, Blundell MP, Cory GO, et al. Two novel activating mutations in the Wiskott-Aldrich syndrome protein result in congenital neutropenia. Blood. 2006;108(7):2182–9.

16

Care of a Toddler with Epistaxis and Bernard-Soulier Syndrome

Melissa J. Rose and
Amanda Jacobson-Kelly

Case Presentation You are called by the emergency department about a 3-year-old girl presenting with a nosebleed. The child's mother reports that the girl has had at least 10 nosebleeds in her life, but this one is the worst she has ever had. Her nose has been bleeding for 6 hours. It will stop when pressure is applied but quickly rebleeds when pressure is removed. The mother also reports that the child frequently has gingival bleeding when brushing her teeth. Neither nosebleeds nor gum bleeding are new symptoms; they have been happening for over a year. The girl has never

M. J. Rose (✉) · A. Jacobson-Kelly
Nationwide Children's Hospital, Division of Pediatric Hematology, Oncology and Bone Marrow Transplant, Columbus, OH, USA

Department of Pediatrics, The Ohio State University College of Medicine, Columbus, OH, USA
e-mail: Melissa.Rose@NationwideChildrens.org;
Amanda.Jacobson@NationwideChildrens.org

seen a hematologist or otolaryngologist for evaluation of nosebleeds, but she has an appointment scheduled in 2 weeks with both specialists. She is otherwise healthy, with normal development, and has never had any surgeries. She has not had any recent illnesses. There is no one in her family with a bleeding disorder.

On exam, she is anxious but overall well-appearing. She is not dysmorphic. She has mild tachycardia but otherwise normal vital signs for age. She has a normal intraoral exam. She oozes from her nose when you remove the nose clamp from her nostrils. You see scattered petechiae on her ankles and around her waist. She has a few small bruises on her shins. Exam is otherwise normal.

A complete blood count (CBC) shows thrombocytopenia (platelets of 70,000/μL). Hemoglobin is also low at 8.5 gm/dL. Of note, the girl had a normal point-of-care hemoglobin 2 days ago, as screening for iron deficiency at her pediatrician's office; she has never had a full CBC obtained until today. White blood cell count and differential are normal. Her blood smear shows thrombocytopenia with giant platelets. Red blood cells appear diminished but are morphologically normal; white blood cells appear morphologically normal as well. A prothrombin time (PT), partial thromboplastin time (PTT), and fibrinogen level are normal.

Multiple-Choice Management Question

What would be the next BEST step in management of this patient?

(a) **Platelet transfusion**
(b) Dexamethasone IV
(c) IVIg
(d) Oral aminocaproic acid

Differential Diagnosis

The differential diagnosis for this child includes immune thrombocytopenia (ITP), an infiltrative bone marrow disease (i.e., leukemia), disseminated intravascular coagulation (DIC), thrombotic thrombocytopenic purpura (TTP), hemolytic uremic syndrome (HUS), or a congenital thrombocytopenia, like gray platelet syndrome, MYH9-related disease, or DiGeorge syndrome-related thrombocytopenia. In this patient, her bleeding symptoms are not new, so this is unlikely to be an acute process, like acute ITP. She is also well-appearing and has no other clinical or laboratory features to suggest HUS, DIC, leukemia, or TTP. Chronic ITP is a possibility, in which you can see few large, but not giant, platelets on a peripheral blood smear, though MPV is typically normal. Also, it would be unusual to have significant prolonged epistaxis causing anemia due to acute blood loss with ITP and a platelet count of 70,000/µL.

In this clinical case, an inherited macrothrombocytopenia is the most likely diagnosis. The patient is otherwise healthy and non-dysmorphic, so DiGeorge syndrome, which is often associated with congenital heart disease, dysmorphic facies, and immunodeficiency, and MYH9-related disease, which is associated with hearing loss, nephritis, and cataracts, are less likely [1, 2]. Additionally, the patient does not have granulocyte inclusions (Dohle-like bodies) on peripheral blood smear, as is often seen in MYH9-related disease, though not required for diagnosis. Therefore, Bernard-Soulier syndrome (BSS) or gray platelet syndrome is the most likely diagnosis. Gray platelet syndrome patients typically have a milder bleeding tendency in comparison to BSS patients. Emergent management for bleeding for either of these conditions would be similar.

In this case, the patient has Bernard-Soulier syndrome (BSS). BSS is an autosomal recessive inherited bleeding tendency also known as hemorrhagiparous thrombocytic dystrophy. It is associated with low platelet counts and giant platelets on blood smear. The defect only affects cells of the megakaryocyte/platelet lineage and therefore is not associated with other cytopenias unless anemia, due to acute and/or chronic blood loss, and iron deficiency is present.

Management Options

Because the patient has an acute drop in hemoglobin and continues to have active bleeding, a platelet transfusion would be the next best step in management. Trying oral aminocaproic acid is also a reasonable option, but it may not stop bleeding quickly enough. An emergent consult to otolaryngology is also an option as they may be able to implement local therapies to stop bleeding.

Platelet Transfusions

Platelet or whole blood transfusions are the best therapeutic measure for correction of uncontrolled bleeding or bleeding prophylaxis prior to surgical procedures. However, repeated exposure to transfused blood products increases risk of alloimmunization and resultant platelet refractoriness. Strategies to reduce alloimmunization include use of leukocyte-reduced products and use of human leukocyte antigen (HLA)-matched donors [3, 4]. HLA typing would not be known in a new emergent situation, but planning for future transfusions by sending a sample for HLA typing is beneficial. Use of platelet apheresis from a single donor can also be helpful to limit donor exposures [5].

Antifibrinolytic Agents

Antifibrinolytic agents, including aminocaproic acid or tranexamic acid, can be beneficial to treat mucosal bleeding and/or help prevent surgical bleeding. They can be adjuncts to other measures. These agents are not effective in all patients with BSS.

DDAVP and rFVIIa

Desmopressin (DDAVP) can also be used to augment hemostasis in the perioperative period. Administration of DDAVP can lead to hyponatremia; thus, fluid intake (both oral and intravenous) must be limited to no more than maintenance during the 24 hour period following DDAVP [5]. rFVIIa is not FDA approved for use in patients with BSS; however, there are case reports of effectiveness of this agent.

Laboratory Findings

On CBC, there will be a small number of very large (giant) platelets. Platelet counts typically range from 20,000 to 100,000/μL, though some patients have low normal platelet counts. Mean platelet volume (MPV) is often unable to be calculated on automated CBC, but will be elevated, if available [6]. A peripheral blood smear will show giant platelets with a rounded shape (Fig. 16.1). Manual counting of platelets may be necessary to accurately assess platelet count, as giant platelets can be falsely identified as lymphocytes with an automated count [4]. Hemoglobin and red blood cell indices should be normal, unless there is a coexisting iron deficiency anemia due to blood loss. White blood cell count and differential should be normal.

Platelet aggregation testing will characteristically reveal an absent response to ristocetin-induced agglutination and a slow response to low, but not high, doses of thrombin. Aggregation responses to adenosine diphosphate and collagen will be normal. When normal plasma is added, there will still be no response to ristocetin (Fig. 16.2). When normal plasma is added to samples from patients with von Willebrand disease, ristocetin-induced agglutination normalizes [4, 7]. On platelet function analysis (PFA-100), closure time will typically be prolonged, but sensitivity is variable depending on the defect, so aggregation studies and/or flow cytometry is needed for confirmation [3].

Flow cytometry will show complete loss of surface CD42b antigen expression (demonstrating a severe deficiency in glycoprotein Ibα (GPIbα)). Other platelet antigens (CD41 and CD61) will be normal [3].

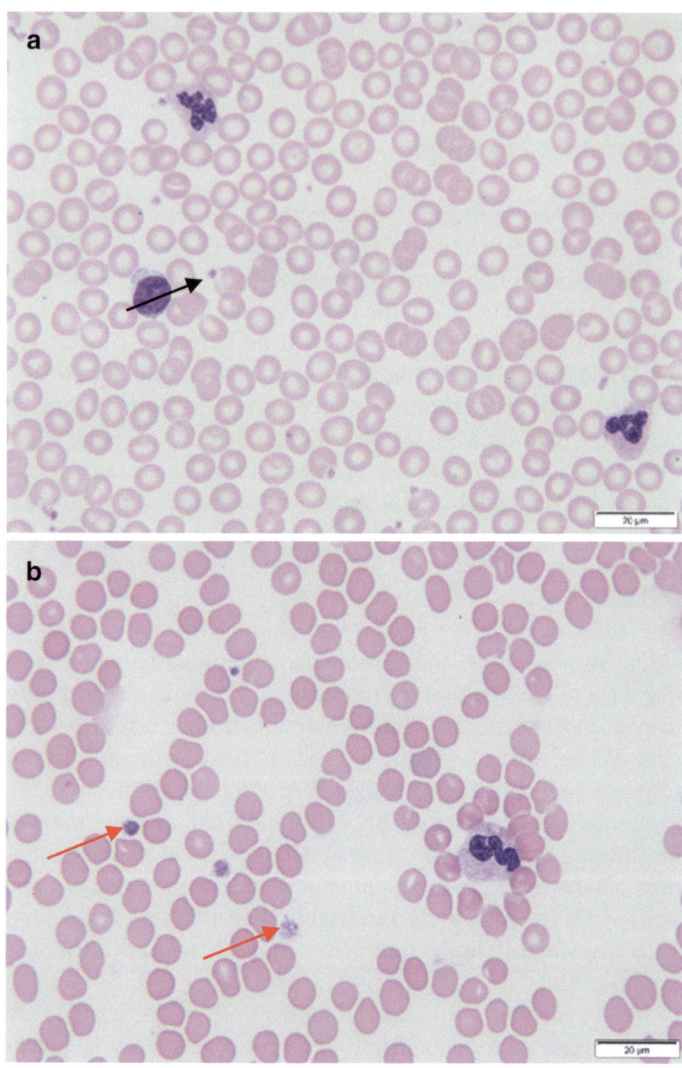

Fig. 16.1 Macrothrombocytopenia in BSS. Panel (**a**) shows a normal peripheral blood smear with normal-sized platelets (black arrow). Panel (**b**) is a peripheral blood smear of a patient with BSS. Macrothrombocytes are shown (red arrows). (Picture provided by Samir B. Kahwash, MD. Department of Pathology and Laboratory Medicine, Nationwide Children's Hospital, Columbus, OH)

16 Care of a Toddler with Epistaxis and Bernard-Soulier Syndrome 177

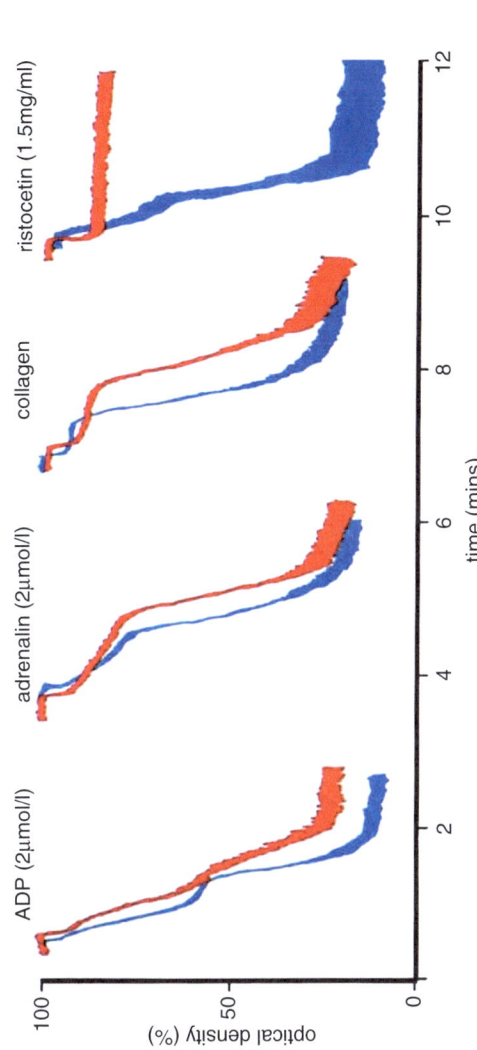

Fig. 16.2 This image demonstrates a classic platelet aggregation tracing in a patient with BSS where the only abnormality is a lack of agglutination with ristocetin. (Used with permission from McGraw-Hill Education)

Epidemiology, Clinical Presentation, and Inheritance/Genetics

Epidemiology

BSS is very rare with an estimated prevalence of <1 in 1,000,000, though the disease is thought to be underreported. In the majority of cases, bleeding symptoms typically start shortly after birth or in early childhood, as was illustrated in our case.

Clinical Presentation

Clinical manifestations typically include mucocutaneous bleeding epistaxis, gingival bleeding particularly after dental extraction, menorrhagia in females, and gastrointestinal bleeding or hemorrhage; these can be significant and potentially life-threatening. Joint bleeding or major hematomas are rare. Severe bleeding following surgical procedures can occur. Bleeding tendency varies significantly between affected individuals [4].

Genetics/Pathophysiology

In patients with BSS, platelets have a defect in a major membrane surface glycoprotein (GP), the GPIb-IX-V complex, composed of four glycoproteins: GPIbα, GPIbβ, GPIX, and GPV [8]. There are a number of mutations in genes encoding for the GPIbα, GPIbβ, and GPIX that have been reported in BSS patients including missense, nonsense, frameshift, and gene deletions. These mutations result in either truncated, unstable, or dysfunctional platelet GPIb-IX-V complex [7].

The GPIb-IX-V complex, also known as the von Willebrand factor (vWF) receptor complex (Fig. 16.3), is located on the surface of platelets and is essential for primary hemostasis, because it initiates platelet adhesion at the sites of vascular injury. Normal adhesion occurs when the subendothelial vWF becomes exposed

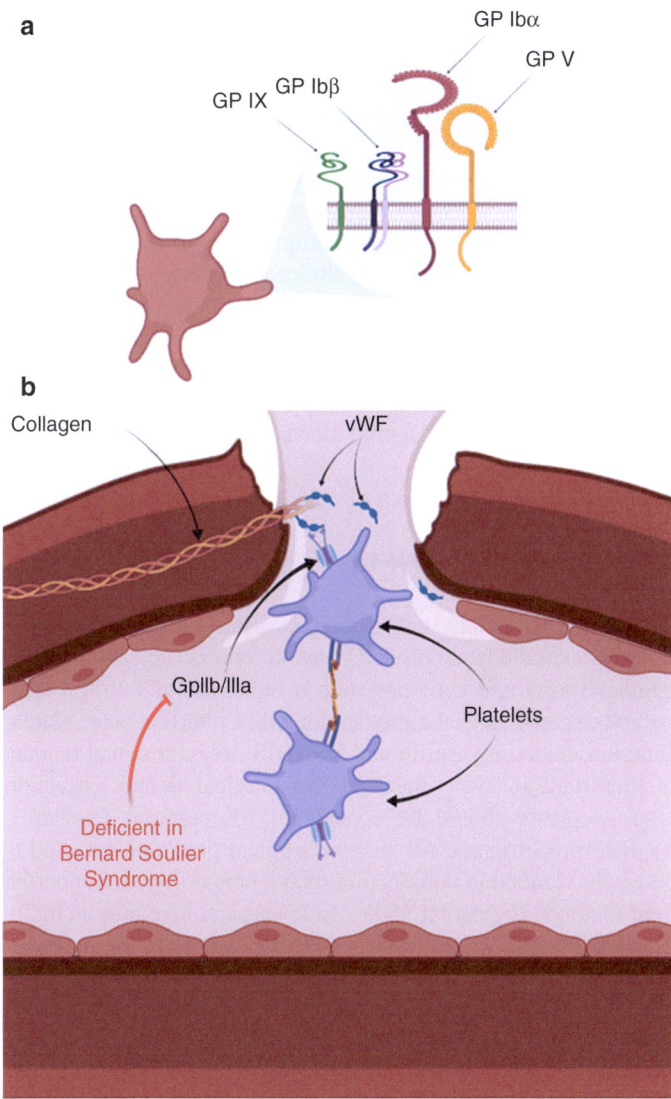

Fig. 16.3 Panel (**a**) demonstrates GPIb-IX-V complex showing GP1bα, GPIbβ, GPIX, and GPV subunits that constitute the complex on platelet surface. The GPIb-IX-V complex's principal function is to initiate arrest of platelets by binding to von Willebrand factor at exposed site of vascular injury. BSS-related dysfunction in this process thus results in impaired primary hemostasis. Panel (**b**) is a schematic of this process. (Both panels were created by Brian Tullius, MD, a fellow physician at Nationwide Children's, using BioRender)

at sites of vascular injury allowing the extracellular domain of GPIbα to bind [4, 8]. Essentially, the GPIb-IX-V complex's principal function is to initiate arrest of platelets at the site of injury [9]. BSS-related dysfunction in this process thus results in impaired primary hemostasis.

As mentioned previously, BSS typically demonstrates an autosomal recessive inheritance pattern. However, there are some patients with heterozygous mutations who have mild macrothrombocytopenia, little to no clinical bleeding symptoms, and normal platelet function [8, 10, 11]. The chromosomal region involved in patients with DiGeorge syndrome (22q11 deletion) contains the gene for one of the four subunits of the GPIb-IX-V complex. Thus, patients with DiGeorge syndrome can have macrothrombocytopenia and a mild bleeding tendency similar to BSS carriers [1].

Outcomes and Follow-Up

In addition to management strategies listed previously, patients with BSS should be counseled to avoid trauma (i.e., avoidance of contact sports and activities with a high risk of falling). Also, patients should not take medications that interfere with platelet function, including aspirin and NSAIDS. Regular dental hygiene is important to avoid the need for surgical dental extraction. Contraceptives should be considered for pubertal females to mediate menorrhagia. All elective surgical procedures should be carefully planned in conjunction with a hematologist. Supportive care methods to prevent and/or treat surgical bleeding including platelet transfusion and use of DDAVP or rFVIIa are described above. In very rare cases in which patients have recurrent life-threatening bleeding, a hematopoietic stem cell transplant can be considered [12]. Patients are typically followed by a hematologist throughout their life. Screening for iron deficiency should be performed regularly, as BSS patients are at risk for iron deficiency due to bleeding, similar to other patients with inherited bleeding disorders. Patients can live a relatively normal life with good education, avoidance of trauma, and adequate specialty care [4].

Clinical Pearls and Pitfalls
- BSS is a rare autosomal recessive macrothrombocytopenia.
- BSS can be difficult to diagnosis based on clinical manifestations alone and thus is often misdiagnosed as ITP. It is important to properly identify BSS, as treatment for ITP including steroids, IVIG, and splenectomy would not be helpful and may even be harmful in BSS.
- On platelet aggregation testing, patients with BSS will have no aggregation with ristocetin but will have normal responses to all other agonists. Aggregation to ristocetin will not normalize with the addition of normal plasma, as it does in von Willebrand disease.
- Manual counting of platelets is often needed to accurately assess platelet count, as giant platelets can be falsely identified as lymphocytes with an automated count.
- Because BSS is both a quantitative and functional disorder of platelets, patients will have bleeding symptoms that are more severe than would be expected for their degree of thrombocytopenia.
- For management of acute, life-threatening hemorrhage, platelet transfusion is the first line of management. However, it is important to remember that patients with BSS are at risk for alloimmunization from platelet transfusions.

References

1. Van Geet C, Devriendt K, Eyskens B, Vermylen J, Hoylaerts MF. Velocardiofacial syndrome patients with a heterozygous chromosome 22q11 deletion have giant platelets. Pediatr Res. 1998;44(4):607–11.
2. Balduini CL, Pecci A, Savoia A. Recent advances in the understanding and management of MYH9-related inherited thrombocytopenias. Br J Haematol. 2011;154(2):161–74.

3. Pham A, Wang J. Bernard-Soulier syndrome: an inherited platelet disorder. Arch Pathol Lab Med. 2007;131(12):1834–6.
4. Lanza F. Bernard-Soulier syndrome (hemorrhagiparous thrombocytic dystrophy). Orphanet J Rare Dis. 2006;1:46.
5. Seligsohn U. Treatment of inherited platelet disorders. Haemophilia. 2012;18(Suppl 4):161–5.
6. Noris P, Klersy C, Gresele P, et al. Platelet size for distinguishing between inherited thrombocytopenias and immune thrombocytopenia: a multicentric, real life study. Br J Haematol. 2013;162(1):112–9.
7. Andrews RK, Berndt MC. Bernard-Soulier syndrome: an update. Semin Thromb Hemost. 2013;39(6):656–62.
8. Savoia A, Pastore A, De Rocco D, et al. Clinical and genetic aspects of Bernard-Soulier syndrome: searching for genotype/phenotype correlations. Haematologica. 2011;96(3):417–23.
9. Lopez JA, Andrews RK, Afshar-Kharghan V, Berndt MC. Bernard-Soulier syndrome. Blood. 1998;91(12):4397–418.
10. Bragadottir G, Birgisdottir ER, Gudmundsdottir BR, et al. Clinical phenotype in heterozygote and biallelic Bernard-Soulier syndrome–a case control study. Am J Hematol. 2015;90(2):149–55.
11. Savoia A, Balduini CL, Savino M, et al. Autosomal dominant macrothrombocytopenia in Italy is most frequently a type of heterozygous Bernard-Soulier syndrome. Blood. 2001;97(5):1330–5.
12. Locatelli F, Rossi G, Balduini C. Hematopoietic stem-cell transplantation for the Bernard-Soulier syndrome. Ann Intern Med. 2003;138(1):79.

Part V

Platelet Dysfunctions

Caring for an Infant with Heelstick Bleeding

17

Gary M. Woods and Riten Kumar

Case Presentation The nursery calls about a 2-day-old, 3.5 kg, male infant with prolonged bleeding following a heelstick that was performed to obtain his newborn screening labs. The child was born full-term via spontaneous vaginal delivery. He received his vitamin K as well as his hepatitis B vaccine without complications. His physical exam and vital signs are normal for age. Although there is no family history of a diagnosed bleeding disorder, the mother reports that she and the infant's father are first-degree cousins.

G. M. Woods
Division of Hematology/Oncology/BMT, Children's Healthcare of Atlanta, Atlanta, GA, USA

Department of Pediatrics, Emory University School of Medicine, Atlanta, GA, USA
e-mail: gary.woods@choa.org

R. Kumar (✉)
Nationwide Children's Hospital, Division of Pediatric Hematology, Oncology and Bone Marrow Transplant, Columbus, OH, USA

Department of Pediatrics, The Ohio State University College of Medicine, Columbus, OH, USA
e-mail: riten.kumar@nationwidechildrens.org

© Springer Nature Switzerland AG 2020
A. L. Dunn et al. (eds.), *Pediatric Bleeding Disorders*,
https://doi.org/10.1007/978-3-030-31661-7_17

Multiple-Choice Management Question

You are concerned that this child may have an inherited bleeding disorder. Your initial evaluation should include:

A. Prothrombin time (PT)
B. Activated partial thromboplastin time (aPTT)
C. Complete blood count (CBC)
D. **All of the above**

Differential Diagnosis

The differential diagnosis for this infant would include hemophilia; rare coagulation factor deficiencies; congenital platelet function defects like Glanzmann thrombasthenia (GT); congenital thrombocytopenias like Bernard-Soulier syndrome, MYH9-related disorders, Wiskott-Aldrich syndrome, etc; neonatal alloimmune thrombocytopenia; and severe von Willebrand disease.

Introduction

Glanzmann thrombasthenia is an autosomal recessive bleeding disorder with an estimated incidence of 1 per million, which may increase to 1 in 200,000 in areas of high consanguinity [1–3]. In 1918, Dr. Eduard Glanzmann first described a bleeding diathesis characterized by a normal platelet count, with slow or absent clot retraction and a prolonged bleeding time, and termed it *Hereditäre hämorrhagische Thrombasthenie*. GT occurs secondary to mutations in the *ITGA2B* (GPIIb) and *ITGB3* (GPIIIa) genes located on chromosome 17, resulting in a quantitative deficiency or a qualitative defect in the platelet membrane glycoprotein GPIIb/IIIa [4]. Insertions, inversions, deletions, nonsense, missense, and frameshift mutations have all been implicated in GT [5, 6]. The reported list of mutations that cause GT can be found at http://sinaicentral.mssm.edu/

intranet/research/glanzmann [7]. These mutations result in production of platelets that are normal in number, but unable to bind to adhesive proteins, including fibrinogen, fibronectin, vitronectin, and von Willebrand, causing significantly reduced platelet aggregation and thrombus formation [8].

The amount of GPIIb/IIIa expressed on platelet surface may be used to classify GT. Type I has <5%, type II has 5–20%, and variant type GT has >20% expression of GPIIb/IIIa [9]. Of note, a correlation between GPIIb/IIIa expression and bleeding severity has not been shown, and affected individuals in the same family, sharing the same mutation, may have different bleeding phenotypes. An exception to this is the stable, milder bleeding phenotype classically seen with the *C807T* polymorphism in *ITGA2* [10, 11].

Clinical Presentation

Severity of bleeding symptoms can vary significantly between individuals with GT, but seem to improve with age [12, 13]. In a French study of 177 patients with GT, most patients were diagnosed before their 5th birthday, emphasizing the early onset of symptoms. In fact, 7/64 (11%) patients were diagnosed in the neonatal period secondary to diffuse petechial rash. Other bleeding symptoms included menorrhagia (98%), easy bruising (86%), epistaxis (73%), and gingival hemorrhage (55%). Of note, three patients (1%) developed intracranial hemorrhage (ICH), usually in the setting of trauma [10]. These initial observations were recently confirmed in a study from Pakistan where easy bruising, epistaxis, and gingival hemorrhage were the most commonly reported symptoms. 2/164 (1%) patients developed ICH, again in the setting of trauma [14]. Of note, some women may elude diagnosis until menarche and present with significant menorrhagia requiring PRBC transfusion and an increased risk of both primary and secondary postpartum hemorrhage [5, 10]. Gastrointestinal hemorrhage, hematuria, and hemarthrosis have been reported as well [12].

Laboratory Findings

The peripheral blood smear in patients with GT is usually normal, though the platelet count may be at the lower end of the normal range [15]. The PT, aPTT, fibrinogen activity, and von Willebrand testing are typically normal. With normal baseline CBC and coagulation testing, this infant should undergo further investigations, including the platelet function analyzer-100 (PFA-100). Both collagen/epinephrine and collagen/adenosine diphosphate closure times on PFA-100 will be prolonged in GT. While not specific for any particular platelet abnormality, the sensitivity for identifying a patient with GT using the PFA-100 has been reported as high as 97% [16]. Platelet aggregation testing will show markedly decreased or absent platelet aggregation to all agonists, except for ristocetin (Fig. 17.1), and diminished clot retraction may also been seen [17].

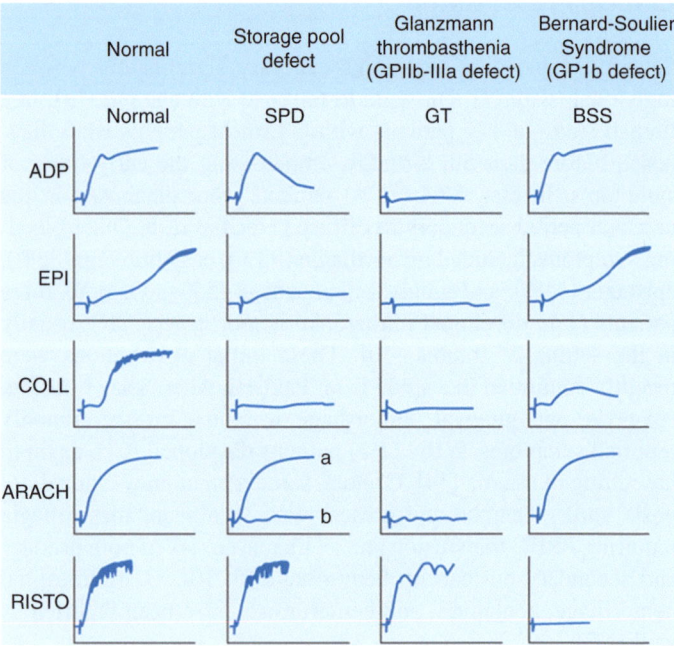

Fig. 17.1 Classic platelet aggregation examples for patients with various platelet function disorders. (Used with permission from source: Jon C. Aster, H. Franklin Bunn. *Pathophysiology of Blood Disorder*, second edition, www.hemonc.mhmedical.com. Copyright © McGraw-Hill Education)

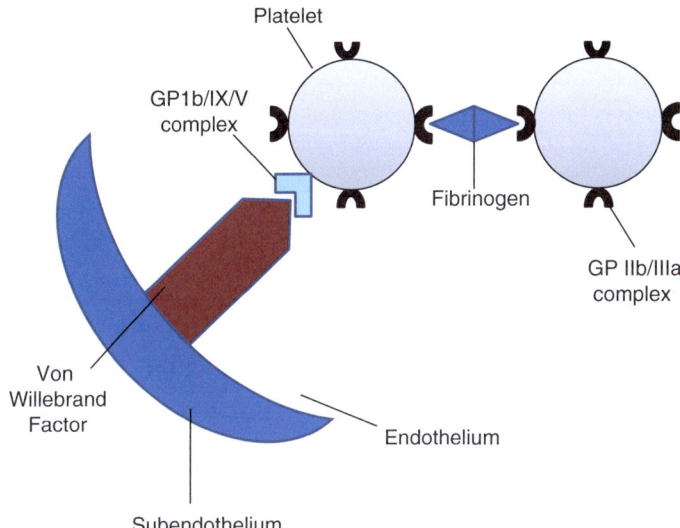

Fig. 17.2 Representation of the GPIIb/IIIa complex

Flow cytometry can be utilized to measure the expression of specific platelet surface receptors using monoclonal antibodies, which in GT would demonstrate significantly decreased expression of the receptor glycoprotein (GP) IIb/IIIa (integrin (ITG) αIIbβ3) (Fig. 17.2) [18]. Direct genomic sequencing of the αIIbβ3 unit may be done to confirm the diagnosis, but is typically not needed [7].

Management Options

Preventative Care

Patients with GT should be managed under the consultation of an experienced hematologist, preferably at a federally funded hemophilia treatment center. Avoiding contact and collision sports, avoiding platelet-altering medications such as NSAIDs and aspirin, and regular dental visits to prevent gingival disease are all recommended to prevent bleeding episodes. Due to the risk with menorrhagia, periodic monitoring for iron deficiency in women should be considered. The use of medical alert apparel is recommended.

Local Control

Mild bleeding symptoms may only require local measures to obtain hemostasis. These can include compression or pressure at the site of bleeding, nasal packing, topical thrombin, or gelatin sponges used as single agents or in combination. Young women with heavy menstrual bleeding may also benefit from exogenous hormonal supplementation. Unfortunately, these measures may not be sufficient to control bleeding symptoms alone, and other methods may need to be utilized in conjunction.

Antifibrinolytics

Antifibrinolytic medications, including ε-aminocaproic acid and tranexamic acid, inhibit plasminogen activation to prevent lysis of formed clots in areas of high fibrinolytic activity. They work well in combination with local control measures to obtain hemostasis during bleeding episodes in GT. Both agents can be given intravenously or orally and are effective in the management of oral mucosal bleeding, menorrhagia, epistaxis and as prophylaxis for minor procedures, including dental extractions [12]. Antifibrinolytic medications should be avoided in the setting of hematuria due to risk of thrombosis in the renal collecting system.

Platelet Transfusions

Platelet transfusions are the standard initial treatment in GT if local measures and/or antifibrinolytics are not effective in controlling bleeding symptoms. Unfortunately, an estimated 30–70% of GT patients will develop alloantibodies to GPIIb/IIIa or HLA isotopes following platelet transfusions [4, 19]. Development of platelet alloimmunization can lead to significant or complete platelet refractoriness. Due to this phenomenon, HLA typing at diagnosis, HLA-matched platelet administration, and regular monitoring for HLA and platelet alloantibodies are recommended [9]. Prior to recombinant factor VIIa (rFVIIa), platelet refractoriness was managed with either plasmapheresis or intravenous immunoglobulin (IVIG) followed by platelet transfusion.

rVIIa

rFVIIa (NovoSeven, Novo Nordisk, Denmark), a recombinant activated human FVII, is approved for perioperative management and treatment of bleeding events in patients with GT who experience platelet refractoriness whether or not a platelet alloantibody is present [7]. Although the mechanism of action is not completely clear, it is believed that rFVIIa, via a tissue factor-independent mechanism, may increase thrombin generation through activation of factors IX and X [19]. It has been shown to be safe and efficacious in treating both bleeding episodes and for perioperative management, but should be administered within 12 hours of symptom onset for optimal hemostasis [9].

rFVIIa may also be utilized to avoid platelet transfusions in the setting of non-life-threatening bleeding events if local control and antifibrinolytics are unsuccessful. In young women, rFVIIa can be used in lieu of platelet transfusions for bleeding events to prevent alloimmunization. This would mitigate the risk of intrauterine death or intracranial hemorrhage from alloantibodies that can be transferred to fetal circulation during pregnancy [19].

Hematopoietic Stem Cell Transplantation (HSCT)

HSCT for GT, though rarely used, remains a curative option for patients with severe platelet refractory GT. Umbilical cord blood, matched unrelated, and HLA-matched sibling donors have all been successfully utilized in HSCT for GT. Sustained engraftment has been shown employing both conventional and reduced-intensity conditioning regimens, and bleeding symptoms have been alleviated even with mixed chimeric engraftment [9].

Gene Therapy

Gene therapy may also offer a treatment option for GT. In both canine and murine models, lentivirus and leukemia retroviruses have been successfully used for gene transfer of CD34+ cells in developing megakaryocytes which resulted in the expression of αIIbβ3 and resolution of GT symptoms. Recent studies have shown success in achieving expression in human megakaryocytes. Although more work is required, gene therapy does offer hope for a GT cure in the future [9].

Outcomes and Follow-Up

Again, patients with GT should be managed under the consultation of an experienced hematologist at a federally funded hemophilia treatment center. Annual follow-up is recommended, with interval clinic visits for spontaneous bleeding events, treatment for injuries, or the development of a perioperative management plan prior to any planned surgical procedure.

> **Clinical Pearls and Pitfalls**
> - GT is inherited in an autosomal recessive fashion, and there is a higher incidence in consanguineous families.
> - Bleeding in GT is quite variable even among family members, and the genotype does not correlate with bleeding symptoms.
> - Bleeding symptoms are generally mucocutaneous and may improve with age.
> - Initial coagulation labs and CBC are generally unremarkable; platelet aggregation studies will show reduced or absent aggregation to all agonists except ristocetin.
> - Local measures and antifibrinolytics are used as first-line therapy, but if bleeding is refractory, rFVIIa should be considered.
> - Platelet transfusion should be reserved for patients truly refractory to first-line therapy, given risk of platelet alloimmunization.

- Platelet alloimmunization following platelet transfusion is a serious concern, so HLA typing at diagnosis, HLA-matched platelet transfusions, and regular monitoring for HLA and platelet antibodies are recommended.
- Care of individuals with GT requires consultation with a hemophilia treatment center.

References

1. Rosas RR, Kurth MH, Sidman J. Treatment and outcomes for epistaxis in children with Glanzmann's thrombasthenia. Laryngoscope. 2010;120(12):2374–7.
2. Newman PJ, et al. The molecular genetic basis of Glanzmann thrombasthenia in the Iraqi-Jewish and Arab populations in Israel. Proc Natl Acad Sci U S A. 1991;88(8):3160–4.
3. Fiore M, et al. Founder effect and estimation of the age of the French Gypsy mutation associated with Glanzmann thrombasthenia in Manouche families. Eur J Hum Genet. 2011;19(9):981–7.
4. Stevens RF, Meyer S. Fanconi and Glanzmann: the men and their works. Br J Haematol. 2002;119(4):901–4.
5. Nurden AT, et al. Glanzmann thrombasthenia: a review of ITGA2B and ITGB3 defects with emphasis on variants, phenotypic variability, and mouse models. Blood. 2011;118(23):5996–6005.
6. Nurden AT, Pillois X, Nurden P. Understanding the genetic basis of Glanzmann thrombasthenia: implications for treatment. Expert Rev Hematol. 2012;5(5):487–503.
7. Nurden AT, Pillois X, Wilcox DA. Glanzmann thrombasthenia: state of the art and future directions. Semin Thromb Hemost. 2013;39(6):642–55.
8. Nurden AT. Glanzmann thrombasthenia. Orphanet J Rare Dis. 2006;1:10.
9. Solh T, Botsford A, Solh M. Glanzmann's thrombasthenia: pathogenesis, diagnosis, and current and emerging treatment options. J Blood Med. 2015;6:219–27.
10. George JN, Caen JP, Nurden AT. Glanzmann's thrombasthenia: the spectrum of clinical disease. Blood. 1990;75(7):1383–95.
11. Fiore M, et al. Clinical utility gene card for: Glanzmann thrombasthenia. Eur J Hum Genet. 2012;20(10):1101.
12. Franchini M, Favaloro EJ, Lippi G. Glanzmann thrombasthenia: an update. Clin Chim Acta. 2010;411(1–2):1–6.

13. Hayward CP, Rao AK, Cattaneo M. Congenital platelet disorders: overview of their mechanisms, diagnostic evaluation and treatment. Haemophilia. 2006;12(Suppl 3):128–36.
14. Iqbal I, Farhan S, Ahmed N. Glanzmann thrombasthenia: a clinicopathological profile. J Coll Physicians Surg Pak. 2016;26(8):647–50.
15. Grainger JD, Thachil J, Will AM. How we treat the platelet glycoprotein defects; Glanzmann thrombasthenia and Bernard Soulier syndrome in children and adults. Br J Haematol. 2018;182(5):621–32.
16. Favaloro EJ. Clinical utility of the PFA-100. Semin Thromb Hemost. 2008;34(8):709–33.
17. Cattaneo M. Light transmission aggregometry and ATP release for the diagnostic assessment of platelet function. Semin Thromb Hemost. 2009;35(2):158–67.
18. Jennings LK, et al. Analysis of human platelet glycoproteins IIb-IIIa and Glanzmann's thrombasthenia in whole blood by flow cytometry. Blood. 1986;68(1):173–9.
19. Bennett JS. Structure and function of the platelet integrin alphaIIbbeta3. J Clin Invest. 2005;115(12):3363–9.

Approach to a Child with Epistaxis and Macrothrombocytopenia

Gary M. Woods and Riten Kumar

Case Presentation A 7-year-old male is referred to the hematology clinic due to recurrent epistaxis and easy bruising. His mother reports that he has always bruised easier than other children and that he has had epistaxis for as long as she can remember. His mother also reports a personal history of epistaxis and is additionally being evaluated for hearing loss. Further examination of the family history reveals that the maternal grandfather also has a history of epistaxis, renal failure requiring dialysis, and hearing loss.

G. M. Woods
Division of Hematology/Oncology/BMT, Children's Healthcare of Atlanta, Atlanta, GA, USA

Department of Pediatrics, Emory University School of Medicine, Atlanta, GA, USA
e-mail: gary.woods@choa.org

R. Kumar (✉)
Nationwide Children's Hospital, Division of Pediatric Hematology, Oncology and Bone Marrow Transplant, Columbus, OH, USA

Department of Pediatrics, The Ohio State University College of Medicine, Columbus, OH, USA
e-mail: riten.kumar@nationwidechildrens.org

Multiple-Choice Management Question

Based on the child's bleeding history and the family history, what would most likely be seen on evaluation of the patient's peripheral blood smear?

A. Microthrombocytopenia
B. **Macrothrombocytopenia and Dohle-like inclusions in the leukoctyes**
C. Macrothrombocytopenia with a light agranular appearance to the platelets

Differential Diagnosis

The differential diagnosis for this case would include the most common inherited bleeding disorders. von Willebrand disease must be considered due to the presumed autosomal dominant inheritance pattern and the mucocutaneous bleeding symptoms reported. Hemophilia and other factor deficiencies may be considered. Congenital platelet defects should also be included in the differential diagnosis as many are inherited in an autosomal dominant fashion, which is consistent with this family's pedigree. The history of mucocutaneous bleeding symptoms with associated sensorineural hearing loss and renal disease all suggest the likely diagnosis of MYH9-related disease (MYH9-RD).

Introduction

MYH9-RD is an autosomal dominant syndrome complex presenting with macrothrombocytopenia and Dohle-like leukocyte inclusion bodies that are present since birth, with a risk of developing nephropathy, sensorineural hearing loss, and presenile cataracts later in life. Dr. Richard May first described leukocyte inclusion bodies in patients with macrothrombocytopenia in 1909. Subsequently, Dr. Robert Hegglin described an autosomal dominant inheritance pattern in a family with macrothrombocytopenia and leukocyte inclusion bodies. This led to use of the term May-Hegglin anomaly [1]. Over the next several decades, three distinct eponyms, namely, Epstein syndrome, Sebastian syndrome, and Fechtner syndrome, were used to describe the association of deafness, cataract, and renal failure with macrothrombocytopenia. In the year 2000, two independent groups confirmed that all these syndromes derive from mutations in the *MYH9* gene, and the term MYH9-RD is now preferred. Located on chromosome 22q12–13, the *MYH9* gene codes for non-muscle myosin heavy chain IIA (NMMHC-IIA), a hetero-hexatetramer that plays an important role in several cellular functions including motility, phagocytosis, and cytokinesis.

Clinical Presentation

Mild to moderate mucocutaneous bleeding, including epistaxis, easy bruising, and heavy menstrual bleeding, are the most common bleeding symptoms reported [1]. Although uncommon, life-threatening bleeding, including intracranial hemorrhage, has been reported [2].

Non-hematologic manifestations of MYH9-RD include nephritis, sensorineural hearing loss, presenile cataracts, and elevated transaminases. In a seminal, cross-sectional study of 108 consecutive patients with MYH9-RD, Pecci and colleagues estimated that approximately 28% of patients experience nephritis, 60% experience sensorineural hearing loss, and 16% develop presenile cataracts. Nephritis and presenile cataracts had a mean age of onset of about 23 years, while sensorineural hearing loss was seen across all ages [3]. Mild to moderate transaminase elevation has been reported in about 50% of cases [4].

Laboratory Findings

Peripheral blood smears in patients with MYH9-RD classically demonstrate macrothrombocytopenia and leukocyte inclusion bodies (Fig. 18.1a). Mean platelet counts can range between 20

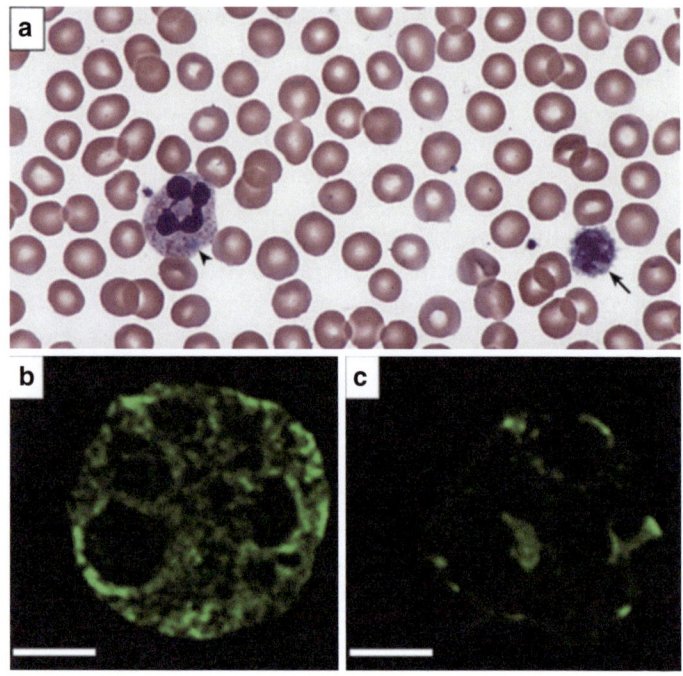

Fig. 18.1 MYH9-RD. (**a**) Peripheral blood smear showing a giant platelet (arrow) and Dohle-like inclusion bodies in a neutrophil (arrowhead) from a patient with MYH9-RD. (**b**) Immunofluorescence microscopy from a blood smear showing normal distribution of NMMHC-IIA in an unaffected patient. (**c**) Multiple cytoplasmic clusters of NMMHC-IIA in a neutrophil from a patient with MYH9-RD. (Reproduced with permission from Kumar et al. [1])

and $130 \times 10^9/L$, and the mean platelet volume (MPV) is typically greater than 12.4 fL [1]. It is important to review the peripheral smear manually. Automated cell counters have been shown to dramatically under report platelet counts, as large platelets can be erroneously counted as red blood cells or leukocytes [3]. Manual cell counts should especially be pursued when leukocytosis is reported.

Dohle-like faint basophilic inclusion bodies can be seen in the cytoplasm of neutrophils. These represent aggregates of NMMHC-IIA. These inclusions have been reported in 40–80% of patients with MYH9-RD [5]. Since these inclusions are not appreciated on peripheral smear of all MYH9-RD patients, the current recommendation is to pursue immunofluorescence staining to detect NMMHC-IIA clusters (Fig. 18.1b, c) [1, 6]. Additionally, genetic testing may be pursued given an evolving insight into the genotype-phenotype correlation. Mutations in the N-terminal, head domain of the heavy chain of the NMMHC-IIA, are typically associated with severe thrombocytopenia, nephritis, and sensorineural hearing loss. In contrast, mutations in the tail domain are associated with hematologic manifestations alone.

Other laboratory workup for MYH9-RD will show a normal prothrombin time (PT), activated partial thromboplastin time (aPTT), and normal von Willebrand antigen and activity testing. Platelet aggregation testing often shows an absent shape change in the aggregation curve due to the associated platelet cytoskeleton changes [6, 7]. The absence of this shape change is not specific to MYH9-RD [6]. Urinalysis may show proteinuria, and serum creatinine may be elevated in patients with renal involvement.

Management Options

Preventative Care

As with other bleeding disorders, avoiding contact and collision sports and platelet-altering medications like nonsteroidal anti-inflammatory drugs and aspirin are prudent to avoid bleeding events [6]. Regular dental visits to prevent gingival disease and use of nasal ointment to reduce epistaxis are recommended. Periodic monitoring for iron deficiency, especially in women with heavy menstrual bleeding, should be considered as significant anemia may further impair already weakened platelet-subendothelial interactions [6].

Local Control

Since most bleeding symptoms are mucocutaneous, local measures of hemostasis control are often sufficient. These can include nasal moisturizers, pressure, and ice.

Desmopressin

Desmopressin, a synthetic analogue of vasopressin, is thought to exert its procoagulant activity by elevating plasma concentrations of both factor VIII and von Willebrand factor. It has been proposed that desmopressin can increase the ability of platelets to adhere to the subendothelial matrix and improve platelet aggregation which can shorten bleeding episodes in patients with inherited platelet disorders [8]. Desmopressin has been shown to be effective in managing certain bleeding symptoms in some patients with MYH9-RD.

Desmopressin can be administered intranasally, intravenously or subcutaneously and may be dosed every 24 hours, but repeated doses in a short interval may result in tachyphylaxis. Side effects are usually mild and may include flushing, tachycardia, and headaches. There is a significant risk for fluid retention that can lead to hyponatremia and seizures following, so fluid restriction for 24 hours after utilization is recommended.

Antifibrinolytics

Antifibrinolytic medications, like tranexamic acid and ε-aminocaproic acid, have also shown to be effective in managing mild to moderate mucocutaneous bleeding in MYH9-RD. They have been utilized effectively in the management of heavy menstrual bleeding in women with MYH9-RD [6].

Platelet Transfusions

If local measures, desmopressin, and antifibrinolytics are not effective at controlling bleeding symptoms, in case of life-threatening bleeding event, or if major surgery is indicated, platelet transfusions should be utilized to obtain hemostasis in patients with MYH9-RD. However, platelet transfusions should be limited if possible due to the risk of developing alloimmunization. It is recommended that HLA-matched platelets be used if possible to prevent this complication.

Outcomes and Follow-Up

Follow-up with an experienced hematologist, at least annually is recommended, but may be more frequent depending on the frequency of bleeding symptoms. Patients with MYH9-RD should also be referred to specialists to ensure adequate screening if non-hematologic symptoms persist [1].

Screening for renal disease beginning soon after diagnosis is critical to help preserve renal function. Urinalysis with urine microalbumin and creatinine studies as well as serum creatinine should be monitored at least annually [9]. Studies have shown that pharmacologic inhibition of the renin-angiotensin system can reduce proteinuria in MYH9-RD [10]. Institution of these therapies at an early stage of renal insufficiency may help slow the progression of this complication in patients with MYH9-RD.

Audiology evaluation should be completed at least every 3 years [9]. Once identified, referral to a hearing specialist should be made, and further follow-up should be at their recommendation. There is no treatment for primary hearing loss; hearing aids and cochlear implants may be beneficial. NMMHC-IIA fixes the cilia of the inner ear in position, so it is recommended to avoid loud noises starting at a young age so ciliary function may be preserved for as long as possible [6].

Ophthalmologic evaluations should be conducted every 3 years until cataracts have been identified. Once identified, referral to an ophthalmologist should be made, and the frequency of follow-up and treatment decisions for further management should be done under the care of the treating ophthalmologist [9].

Clinical Pearls and Pitfalls
- MYH9-RD are characterized by the triad of thrombocytopenia, large platelets, and Dohle-like leukocyte inclusion bodies.
- Mucocutaneous bleeding, including epistaxis, easy bruising, and heavy menstrual bleeding, are the most common bleeding symptoms.

- Local measures, antifibrinolytics, and desmopressin are used as first-line therapy for bleeding events, but if bleeding is refractory, platelet transfusions should be considered.
- Nephritis, sensorineural hearing loss, and presenile cataracts are common non-hematologic manifestations of MYH9-RD.
- Screening for the common non-hematologic complications should be completed regularly, and interventions begun soon after identification.
- Bleeding disorder management of MYH9-RD should be done under the supervision of a hemophilia treatment center.

References

1. Kumar R, Kahr WH. Congenital thrombocytopenia: clinical manifestations, laboratory abnormalities, and molecular defects of a heterogeneous group of conditions. Hematol Oncol Clin North Am. 2013;27(3):465–94.
2. Leung TF, Tsoi WC, Li CK, Chik KW, Shing MM, Yuen PM. A Chinese adolescent girl with Fechtner-like syndrome. Acta Paediatr. 1998;87(6):705–7.
3. Pecci A, Panza E, Pujol-Moix N, et al. Position of nonmuscle myosin heavy chain IIA (NMMHC-IIA) mutations predicts the natural history of MYH9-related disease. Hum Mutat. 2008;29(3):409–17.
4. Pecci A, Biino G, Fierro T, et al. Alteration of liver enzymes is a feature of the MYH9-related disease syndrome. PLoS One. 2012;7(4):e35986.
5. Pecci A, Panza E, De Rocco D, et al. MYH9 related disease: four novel mutations of the tail domain of myosin-9 correlating with a mild clinical phenotype. Eur J Haematol. 2010;84(4):291–7.
6. Althaus K, Greinacher A. MYH9-related platelet disorders. Semin Thromb Hemost. 2009;35(2):189–203.
7. Canobbio I, Noris P, Pecci A, Balduini A, Balduini CL, Torti M. Altered cytoskeleton organization in platelets from patients with MYH9-related disease. J Thromb Haemost. 2005;3(5):1026–35.

8. Cattaneo M. Desmopressin in the treatment of patients with defects of platelet function. Haematologica. 2002;87(11):1122–4.
9. Savoia A, Pecci A. MYH9-related disorders. In: Adam MP, Ardinger HH, Pagon RA, et al, editors. GeneReviews [Internet]. Seattle: University of Washington; 1993–2018. Available from: https://www.ncbi.nlm.nih.gov/books/NBK2689/. 2008 Nov 20 [Updated 2015 July 16].
10. Pecci A, Granata A, Fiore CE, Balduini CL. Renin-angiotensin system blockade is effective in reducing proteinuria of patients with progressive nephropathy caused by MYH9 mutations (Fechtner-Epstein syndrome). Nephrol Dial Transplant. 2008;23(8):2690–2.

19

Recognition and Management of Congenital Platelet Granule Disorders

Gary M. Woods and Riten Kumar

Case Presentation A 14-year-old female is referred to hematology secondary to heavy menstrual bleeding. Menarche occurred at the age of 11 years, and she reports that her menstrual cycles have always lasted greater than 7 days. Additionally, she reports having accidents despite changing her sanitary pads every 2–3 hours on her heaviest days and waking up at night to change pads. There are no other reported bleeding symptoms, and the family denies a history of known bleeding disorders. On exam, you notice that she has oculocutaneous albinism, and when

---

G. M. Woods
Division of Hematology/Oncology/BMT, Children's Healthcare of Atlanta, Atlanta, GA, USA

Department of Pediatrics, Emory University School of Medicine, Atlanta, GA, USA
e-mail: gary.woods@choa.org

R. Kumar (✉)
Nationwide Children's Hospital, Division of Pediatric Hematology, Oncology and Bone Marrow Transplant, Columbus, OH, USA

Department of Pediatrics, The Ohio State University College of Medicine, Columbus, OH, USA
e-mail: riten.kumar@nationwidechildrens.org

inquired about, the family reports that her brother also has this finding. The family also notes that her maternal grandfather had similar skin findings and had respiratory issues develop at a relatively young age. You discover the family immigrated to the United States from Puerto Rico before the patient was born.

Multiple-Choice Management Question

You are concerned based on the history that this patient likely has a defect affecting:

A. **Platelets**
B. Von Willebrand factor
C. Factor VIII
D. Factor X

Differential Diagnosis

von Willebrand disease must be considered in any young woman presenting with menorrhagia. Hemophilia should also be considered as young women who are carriers for FVIII or FIX deficiency may present with heavy menstrual bleeding. Other factor deficiencies may also be considered, especially in specific patient populations. Immune thrombocytopenia may lead to similar findings and should be evaluated for, but the family history suggests an inherited disorder. Inherited platelet function disorders (IPFD) would be of high concern for this patient, especially a platelet storage pool deficiency (PSPD) which may be associated with oculocutaneous albinism in patients with Hermansky-Pudlak syndrome.

Epidemiology, Clinical Findings, and Diagnosis

Platelets consist of three unique types of cytoplasmic storage granules, namely, α-granules, δ-granules, and lysosomes. Of these, α-granules are the largest and most predominant, with

50–80 alpha granules per platelet, while lysosomes and δ-granules are present at about 2, and 3–8 granules per platelet, respectively [1]. α-granule contains numerous proteins involved in hemostasis, including coagulation factors (II, V, and XI), anticoagulant/fibrinolytic proteins (protein S, tissue factor pathway inhibitor, urokinase plasminogen activator (uPA), plasminogen activator inhibitor 1), growth factors, angiogenic factors, and immune modulators. δ-granules contain proaggregatory factors including adenosine diphosphate (ADP), adenosine triphosphate (ATP), and serotonin; lysosomes contain elastase, carboxypeptidase, and collagenase [1].

Platelet granule disorders can arise from a deficiency of any of these granules, most commonly the α- or δ-granules, or from a disorder in the release/secretion of granule contents. Platelet secretion involves a complex process that starts with a platelet-agonist interaction with the platelet via its receptor and continues through granule fusion with the platelet membrane resulting in the release of granule contents. Any defect in this process will result in poor platelet response and activation resulting in a bleeding diathesis [1].

Platelet Storage Pool Deficiency (PSPD)

The term PSPD encompasses a heterogeneous group of disorders that result from a deficiency of either the α-granules or δ-granules or decreased granule content [2]. Often, disorders associated with PSPD are complex and are associated with known syndromes that affect other organ systems [3]. Mild-to-moderate mucocutaneous bleeding is the most common symptom reported.

Delta Granule Storage Pool Deficiency (δ-PSPD)

δ-PSPD is characterized by a lack of platelet δ-granules, which leads to a deficit in platelet aggregation resulting in a bleeding diathesis, which is generally mild to moderate in nature [2]. δ-PSPD is most often associated with mucocutaneous bleeding symptoms, including easy bruising, heavy menstrual bleeding, epistaxis, and bleeding from trauma and surgical challenges [3]. The prothrombin time (PT), activated partial thromboplastin time

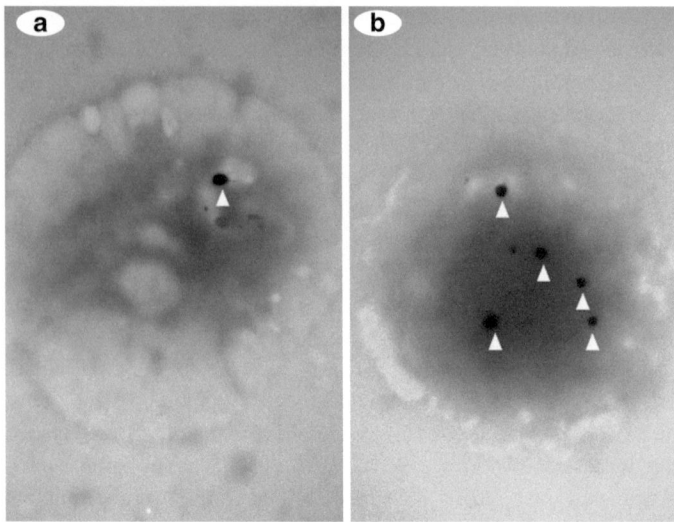

Fig. 19.1 Panel (**a**) shows a platelet EM with only one δ-granule noted. Panel (**b**) shows a normal platelet EM with numerous δ-granules present [5]

(aPTT), and platelet function analyzer-100 (PFA-100) closure times are normal [4]. Platelets are usually normal in number and size. Platelet EM will show a paucity or absence of δ-granules (Fig. 19.1 [5]), and light transmission aggregometry (LTA) results may be variable. δ-PSPD is usually classified as either congenital, including Hermansky-Pudlak and Chediak-Higashi syndromes, or idiopathic inherited δ-PSPD [6].

Hermansky-Pudlak Syndrome

Hermansky-Pudlak syndrome (HPS) is a rare autosomal recessive multisystem disorder, with ten subtypes described in the literature secondary to ten different mutations in the *HPS* gene (*HPS1*-*HPS10*) [7]. Although this disease is rare, it is the most common genetic condition in Puerto Rico, affecting about 1 in every 800 individuals, with the *HPS1* mutation the most common causative mutation [8].

Mutations in *HPS*-associated genes result in defects in the intracellular protein trafficking and in the biogenesis of lysosomes and dense granules. Typical phenotypic presentation includes oculocutaneous albinism characterized by hypopigmentation of the skin and hair, characteristic eye findings, and reduced dense granules on platelet electron microscopy. Depending on the subtype, patients may additionally develop pulmonary fibrosis, nystagmus, early-onset cataracts, granulomatous colitis, neutropenia, and immunodeficiency. Pulmonary fibrosis can be seen in HPS1 and HPS4 mutations and typically develops in the third and fourth decade of life, whereas nystagmus, cataracts, and granulomatous colitis are associated with an HPS1 mutation [9]. HPS2 mutations may have an associated neutropenia and immunodeficiency [10].

Chediak-Higashi Syndrome

Chediak-Higashi syndrome (CHS) is a rare autosomal recessive disorder characterized by severe immunodeficiency, recurrent pyogenic infections, oculocutaneous albinism, progressive neurological dysfunction, and δ-PSPD. The disorder results from frameshift or nonsense mutation in the *CHS1/LYST* gene which codes for a vesicle trafficking regulatory protein. Patients are typically affected by recurrent bacterial infections secondary to severe immunodeficiency and an accelerated lymphohistiocytic proliferation in multiple organs that is usually fatal in the first decade of life [3]. The only cure is a hematopoietic stem cell transplant (HSCT). Neurological problems including ataxia, weakness, sensory deficits, and progressive neurodegeneration may be seen in 10–15% of patients who survive early childhood with HSCT [11].

The classic laboratory findings showed decreased and/or irregular δ-granules on EM, and LTA will show decreased response to all agonists. Large peroxidase-positive granules in the cytoplasm of the neutrophils are pathognomic of CHS.

Idiopathic δ-PSPD

δ-PSPD may not be associated without other clinical characteristics and can be an isolated finding. Idiopathic δ-PSPD describes a large cohort of patients with substantial variability in bleeding severity, as well as the laboratory findings. LTA testing may show decreased or absent aggregation to any of the agonists. Of note, however, platelet EM findings do not always correlate with LTA findings underscoring the inherent difficulty in diagnosing this condition [12].

Alpha Granule Storage Pool Deficiency (α-PSPD)

α-PSPD is generally associated with syndromes that have specific clinical findings as well as a deficiency in α-platelet granules. Alpha platelet granules are known to contain many proteins, including factor V, fibrinogen, von Willebrand factor, and P-selectin, among others, that assist in hemostasis. Bleeding diathesis is usually mild to moderate and mucocutaneous in nature. The PT and aPTT are unaffected; PFA-100 results are variable. Macrothrombocytopenia is often present.

Gray Platelet Syndrome (GPS)

GPS is a rare, predominantly autosomal recessive bleeding disorder caused by mutations in the *NBEAL2* gene, although autosomal dominant inheritance patterns involving the *GF1B* have been described [7]. *NBEAL2* encodes a protein containing a BEACH (beige and Chediak-Higashi syndrome) domain that is involved in vesicular trafficking and is critical for the development of α-granules. Bleeding symptoms range from mild mucocutaneous bleeding, to postsurgical hemorrhage and fatal menorrhagia. Thrombocytopenia is moderate and tends to correlate negatively with age, such that older patients tend to have lower platelet counts [13]. Myelofibrosis with associated splenomegaly is seen in more than 80% of patients.

The blood smear in patients with GPS usually reveals thrombocytopenia with large and misshapen platelets that are gray in color due to absence of basophilic staining of the α-granules (Fig. 19.2). Platelet EM shows complete absence of α-granules, with normal dense granules and lysosomes. Platelet aggregation testing has been shown to be quite variable, ranging from normal to defects in one or more of the agonists, including lack of response to collagen [3].

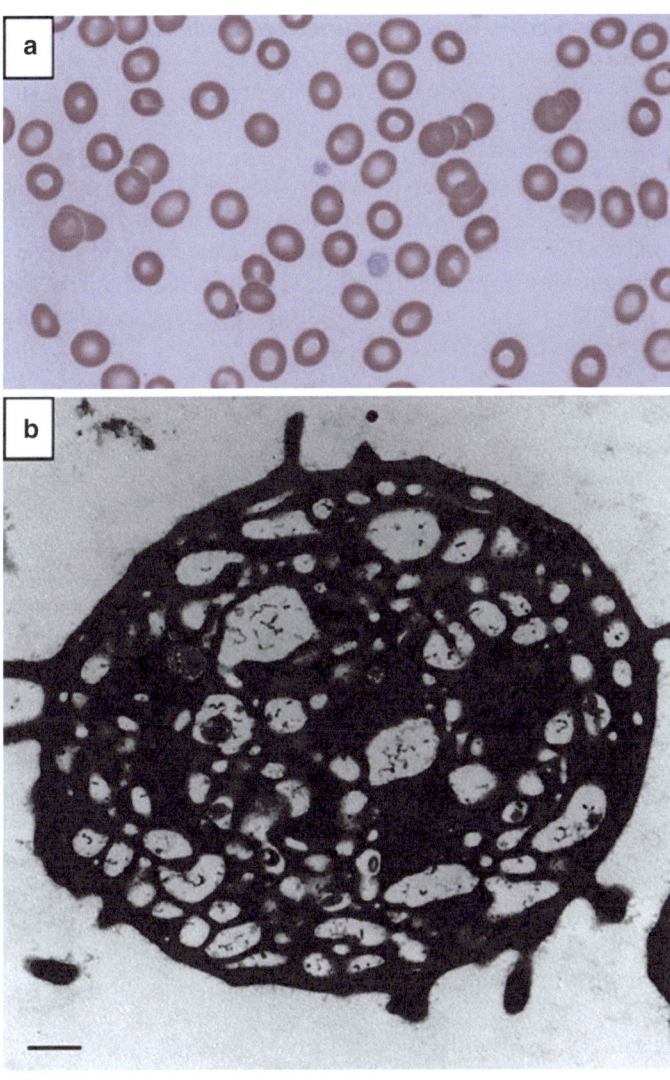

Fig. 19.2 Large gray-appearing platelets on Wright-Giemsa stain in GPS (Panel **a**). Absent alpha granules and increased vacuoles on platelet EM in GPS (Panel **b**) [13]

Arthrogryposis-Renal Dysfunction-Cholestasis (ARC) Syndrome

ARC syndrome is a rare fatal, autosomal recessive disorder that is associated with a deficiency in platelet α-granules. It is a multisystem disorder associated with joint contractures, renal tubular dysfunction, and cholestasis, as well as severe failure to thrive and central nervous system malformations. It is caused by mutations in *VPS33B* or *VIPAR* genes and is usually identified by the known distinguishing features. Most affected patients die within the first year of life [3, 14]. Platelet EM will show an absence of platelet α-granules and δ-granules [15].

X-Linked Thrombocytopenia (With or Without Dyserythropoietic Anemia)

Germline mutations in GATA1 located on Xp11.23, a gene that encodes a zinc finger DNA-binding transcription factor involved in the development of hematopoietic stem cells, cause an X-linked recessive macrothrombocytopenia with our without dyserythropoietic anemia [7, 16]. Clinically significant mucocutaneous bleeding has been reported as early as the neonatal period, as well as associations with cryptorchidism, splenomegaly, neutropenia, beta thalassemia, and a congenital erythropoietic porphyria [7, 13]. The thrombocytopenia is generally severe, platelet aggregation results are variable, but reduced aggregation to collagen has been described, and decreased or absent α-granules on EM have been reported [13, 17]. Supportive care with transfusions of platelets and red blood cells is the mainstay for management, but HSCT has been successful in curing severe cases [13].

Platelet Release Disorders

Platelet release disorder describes a heterogeneous group of disorders that have a defect in the release of the granule content. This can be due to a true secretion deficit or increased degradation of platelet granule contents. The most common reported bleeding diathesis is mucocutaneous in nature and is mild to moderate in severity. Platelet aggregation testing will be variable, and decreased aggregation to any agonist can be seen. PFA-100 can also be variable, but prolongation to both collagen/epinephrine and collagen/ADP can be seen, while the PT and aPTT are unaffected.

Paris-Trousseau/Jacobsen Syndrome

Paris-Trousseau or Jacobsen syndrome is an autosomal dominant macrothrombocytopenia with a subpopulation of platelets demonstrating giant fused α-granules that stain red on the Wright-Giemsa stain. These platelets are unable to release the contents of their α-granules upon stimulation [18]. This syndrome is caused by constitutional deletions in the distal portion of chromosome 11, including the *FLI1* locus, and is associated with other congenital features, including craniofacial abnormalities, cardiac anomalies, and mental retardation [7]. Mucocutaneous bleeding is the most common, and the bleeding diathesis is mild to moderate in nature.

Parris-Trousseau or Jacobsen syndrome is usually associated with moderate thrombocytopenia, with a trend toward improvement in platelet count later in life [7]. On peripheral blood smear, giant α-granules can be seen within the large platelets, and platelet EM can confirm the presence of fused granules (Fig. 19.3) [19].

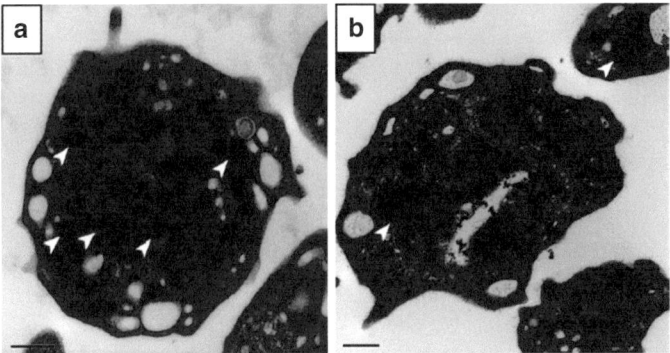

Fig. 19.3 Platelet EM of normal platelet (Panel **a**) with platelet EM showing giant alpha granules (arrow head) in Paris-Trousseau (Jacobsen) syndrome (Panel **b**) [13]

Quebec Platelet Disorder (QPD)

QPD is a very rare autosomal dominant bleeding disorder characterized by delayed-onset bleeding. It is caused by a *PLAU* gene tandem duplication [20]. The *PLAU* gene encodes the uPA protein, and the tandem duplication results in overexpression of uPA in the platelet α-granules. The overexpression of uPA leads to degradation of many platelet α-granule proteins, including factor V and P-selectin, and to enhanced clot lysis secondary to increased uPA presence at the location of freshly formed hemostatic plugs [3, 7]. Interestingly, antifibrinolytic medications, like ε-aminocaproic acid and tranexamic acid, are more effective in obtaining hemostasis than platelet transfusions in QPD, possibly due to the large volume of uPA released upon activation [3]. Exceptionally abnormal aggregation to epinephrine can be seen on platelet aggregation testing [21].

Management Options

Preventative Care

Due to the difficulty in diagnosis and rarity of these conditions, the care of patients with PSPD and platelet release disorders should be managed by an experienced hematologist. Preventative measures to reduce the risk of bleeding are similar to that of other mild bleeding disorders: avoidance of contact sports, avoiding platelet-altering medications, regular dental visits to prevent the development of gingival disease, and periodic iron deficiency screening for patients experiencing heavy menstrual bleeding or frequent epistaxis.

Local Control

Generally, the bleeding symptoms are mild, so local control may be adequate at obtaining hemostasis. Local measures include local compression/pressure, nasal packing, nasal cauterization, topical thrombin, or gauze soaked in antifibrinolytic medications, and these can be used in isolation or combination. Antifibrinolytic mouthwash may help control gingival bleeding, and exogenous hormonal supplementation may benefit young women with heavy menstrual bleeding.

Antifibrinolytics

Tranexamic acid and ε-aminocaproic acid are antifibrinolytic medications that inhibit plasminogen activation. This prevents lysis of formed clots in areas of high fibrinolytic activity. They are effective at controlling mucocutaneous bleeding, including epistaxis, oral mucosal bleeding, and heavy menstrual bleeding. These can be given intravenously and orally or used as a mouthwash to control local gingival bleeding. Avoid the use of antifibrinolytic medications in the setting of hematuria due to risk of thrombosis in the renal collecting system.

Desmopressin

Patients with PSPD and platelet release disorders respond to desmopressin, and it should be considered when local measures and antifibrinolytics alone are ineffective at obtaining hemostasis [3]. Evidence supporting the correction of the bleeding time to indicate efficacy is limited, and thus, effect must be judged by clinical response [3]. It can be administered intravenously, subcutaneously, or as an intranasal medication. Although its exact imapct on platelet function in PSPD is not defined, it has been suggested that desmopressin improves the platelet ability to adhere to subendothelial matrices and improve platelet aggregation in inherited platelet disorders [22]. Desmopressin should only be dosed every 24 hours, but generally not more than 2 days in a row and no more than three doses in a week. Repeated doses result in tachyphylaxis resulting in a decreased responsiveness. Fluid restriction for 24 hours following administration is required to avoid fluid retention that can lead to hyponatremia and seizures.

Platelet Transfusions

Platelet transfusions should be utilized if desmopressin, antifibrinolytics, and local measures are ineffective at obtaining hemostasis or if there is a life-threatening bleeding event. Perioperative transfusions may be required for significant surgical procedures as well. Platelet transfusions should be limited due to the complications associated with all transfusions as well as the risk for developing alloimmunization. It is custom to HLA-type patients that may require frequent platelet transfusions and provide HLA-selected platelets to prevent this complication, unless this would cause a significant delay in management and compromise the patient's clinical course [3].

Outcomes and Follow-Up

Due to the complexity in diagnosis and management of patients with PSPD and platelet release disorders, the treatment should be managed under the care of an experienced hematologist at a federally funded hemophilia treatment center. Generally, annual follow-up is all that is required unless there are acute bleeding events that require management beyond local control measures or for the perioperative management of a planned surgical procedure. Patients with associated clinical syndromes should be referred to appropriate consultants to aid in the monitoring and management of the accompanying complications.

> **Clinical Pearls and Pitfalls**
> - PSPD and platelet release disorders are a heterogeneous group of disorders that results from a deficiency or absence of the α-granules or δ-granules or a defect in granule secretion.
> - Many of these conditions may be associated with specific clinical syndromes.
> - The most common bleeding is mucocutaneous, and it is generally mild to moderate in severity.

- Platelet transfusions should only be considered under specific circumstances if local control and other treatment options are unable to obtain hemostasis.
- Platelet alloimmunization following platelet transfusion is a serious concern, so HLA typing at diagnosis, HLA-matched platelet transfusions, and regular monitoring for HLA and platelet antibodies are recommended.
- Individuals with PSPD and platelet release disorders require consultation with a hemophilia treatment center.

References

1. Dorgalaleh A, Tabibian S, Shamsizadeh M. Inherited platelet function disorders (IPFDs). Clin Lab. 2017;63(1):1–13.
2. Simon D, Kunicki T, Nugent D. Platelet function defects. Haemophilia. 2008;14(6):1240–9.
3. Bolton-Maggs PH, Chalmers EA, Collins PW, et al. A review of inherited platelet disorders with guidelines for their management on behalf of the UKHCDO. Br J Haematol. 2006;135(5):603–33.
4. Sladky JL, Klima J, Grooms L, Kerlin BA, O'Brien SH. The PFA-100 (R) does not predict delta-granule platelet storage pool deficiencies. Haemophilia. 2012;18(4):626–9.
5. Woods GM, Pillay Smiley N, Stanek J, Kahwash S, Kerlin BA, O'Brien SH. Variation in platelet delta granules over time in young women undergoing evaluation for heavy menstrual bleeding. Pediatr Dev Pathol. 2019;22(2):123–7.
6. Selle F, James C, Tuffigo M, et al. Clinical and laboratory findings in patients with delta-storage pool disease: a case series. Semin Thromb Hemost. 2017;43(1):48–58.
7. Sharma R, Perez Botero J, Jobe SM. Congenital disorders of platelet function and number. Pediatr Clin North Am. 2018;65(3):561–78.
8. Witkop CJ, Nunez Babcock M, Rao GH, et al. Albinism and Hermansky-Pudlak syndrome in Puerto Rico. Bol Asoc Med P R. 1990;82(8):333–9.
9. Brantly M, Avila NA, Shotelersuk V, Lucero C, Huizing M, Gahl WA. Pulmonary function and high-resolution CT findings in patients with an inherited form of pulmonary fibrosis, Hermansky-Pudlak syndrome, due to mutations in HPS-1. Chest. 2000;117(1):129–36.
10. Fontana S, Parolini S, Vermi W, et al. Innate immunity defects in Hermansky-Pudlak type 2 syndrome. Blood. 2006;107(12):4857–64.

11. Mathis S, Cintas P, de Saint-Basile G, Magy L, Funalot B, Vallat JM. Motor neuronopathy in Chediak-Higashi syndrome. J Neurol Sci. 2014;344(1–2):203–7.
12. Woods GM, Kudron EL, Davis K, Stanek J, Kerlin BA, O'Brien SH. Light transmission aggregometry does not correlate with the severity of delta-granule platelet storage pool deficiency. J Pediatr Hematol Oncol. 2016;38(7):525–8.
13. Kumar R, Kahr WH. Congenital thrombocytopenia: clinical manifestations, laboratory abnormalities, and molecular defects of a heterogeneous group of conditions. Hematol Oncol Clin North Am. 2013;27(3):465–94.
14. Zhou Y, Zhang J. Arthrogryposis-renal dysfunction-cholestasis (ARC) syndrome: from molecular genetics to clinical features. Ital J Pediatr. 2014;40:77.
15. Nurden AT, Nurden P. Should any genetic defect affecting alpha-granules in platelets be classified as gray platelet syndrome? Am J Hematol. 2016;91(7):714–8.
16. Calligaris R, Bottardi S, Cogoi S, Apezteguia I, Santoro C. Alternative translation initiation site usage results in two functionally distinct forms of the GATA-1 transcription factor. Proc Natl Acad Sci U S A. 1995;92(25):11598–602.
17. Freson K, Matthijs G, Thys C, et al. Different substitutions at residue D218 of the X-linked transcription factor GATA1 lead to altered clinical severity of macrothrombocytopenia and anemia and are associated with variable skewed X inactivation. Hum Mol Genet. 2002;11(2):147–52.
18. Breton-Gorius J, Favier R, Guichard J, et al. A new congenital dysmegakaryopoietic thrombocytopenia (Paris-Trousseau) associated with giant platelet alpha-granules and chromosome 11 deletion at 11q23. Blood. 1995;85(7):1805–14.
19. Favier R, Jondeau K, Boutard P, et al. Paris-Trousseau syndrome: clinical, hematological, molecular data of ten new cases. Thromb Haemost. 2003;90(5):893–7.
20. Paterson AD, Rommens JM, Bharaj B, et al. Persons with Quebec platelet disorder have a tandem duplication of PLAU, the urokinase plasminogen activator gene. Blood. 2010;115(6):1264–6.
21. Hayward CP, Rivard GE, Kane WH, et al. An autosomal dominant, qualitative platelet disorder associated with multimerin deficiency, abnormalities in platelet factor V, thrombospondin, von Willebrand factor, and fibrinogen and an epinephrine aggregation defect. Blood. 1996;87(12):4967–78.
22. Cattaneo M. Desmopressin in the treatment of patients with defects of platelet function. Haematologica. 2002;87(11):1122–4.

Index

A
Acquired bone marrow suppression/failure, 142
Acquired von Willebrand disease (AVWD)
  case history, 127, 128
  clinical presentation, 128
  differential diagnosis, 130, 132
  epidemiology, 129
  immune-mediated pathologies, 133
  immune-related mechanisms, 130
  laboratory evaluation, 132
  management, 133–135
  pathophysiology, 130, 131
  treatment outcomes and follow-up, 135, 136
Alpha-granule storage pool deficiency (α-PSPD), 210
American Society of Hematology guidelines, 154
Arthrogryposis-renal dysfunction-cholestasis syndrome (ARC), 212

B
Bernard-Soulier syndrome (BSS)
  antifibrinolytic agents, 174
  case history, 171, 172
  clinical manifestations, 178
  desmopressin (DDAVP), 174, 175
  differential diagnosis, 172, 173
  epidemiology, 178
  genetics/pathophysiology, 178–180
  laboratory findings, 175–177
  platelet transfusions, 174
  rFVIIa, 174, 175
  treatment outcomes and follow-up, 180

C
Chediak-Higashi syndrome (CHS), 209
Concizumab, 21

D
Delta-granule storage pool deficiency (δ-PSPD), 207–208
DiGeorge syndrome, 173

E
Emicizumab, 21

F

Factor VII deficiency
  antifibrinolytic agents, 63
  case history, 59
  clinical manifestations, 62
  coagulation inhibitors, 62
  diagnosis, 61
  differential diagnosis, 60
  epidemiology, 62
  genetic diagnosis, 61
  laboratory findings, 60
  multi-disciplinary clinics, 63
  Seven Treatment Evaluations Registry (STER), 63
  therapeutic options, 63
Factor XI deficiency
  case history, 65
  clinical manifestations, 67
  clinical outcomes, 69
  diagnosis and assessment, 66
  differential diagnoses, 66
  follow-up, 69
  laboratory findings, 66
  laboratory testing, 68
  management options, 68, 69
  mutation subtypes, 68
  prevalence, 68
Factor XIII deficiency
  activated factor XIII (fXIII-A_2*), 73
  A-subunits, 73
  biochemistry, 75
  B-subunits, 73
  case history, 71
  diagnostic algorithm, 74
  differential diagnosis, 72
  fibrinolysis inhibitor, 76
  laboratory findings, 73
  management options, 76, 77
  physiologic function, 74
  prevalence, 76
  treatment outcomes and follow-up, 77, 78
Fibrinogen disorders
  antifibrinolytics, 55
  case history, 51
  clinical manifestations, 52, 53
  concomitant anticoagulant therapy, 57
  differential diagnosis, 52
  epidemiology and inheritance, 55
  laboratory diagnosis, 53, 55
  laboratory findings, 52
  replacement therapy, 55
  topical treatments, 55
Fitusiran, 21

G

Glanzmann thrombasthenia (GT)
  anti-fibrinolytic medications, 190
  bleeding severity, 187
  case history, 185
  clinical presentation, 187
  differential diagnosis, 186
  GBIIb/IIIa expression, 187
  gene therapy, 192
  hematopoietic stem cell transplantation (HSCT), 191
  incidence, 186
  initial evaluation, 186
  laboratory findings, 188, 189
  local control, 190
  platelet transfusions, 190, 191
  preventative care, 189
  treatment outcomes and follow-up, 192
Gray platelet syndrome (GPS), 210–212

H

Hematopoietic stem cell transplant (HCST), 164
Hemophilia A
  activated prothrombin complex concentrate, 19

antifibrinolytic therapy, 9
bleeding manifestations, 6
case history, 13
comprehensive care, 9
concizumab, 21
diagnosis and assessment, 5, 6, 16
differential diagnosis, 4, 14
emicizumab, 19, 21
factor VIII inhibitor by-passing activity, 19
fitusuran, 21
FVIII replacement, 9
genetics, 7
immune tolerance therapy (ITT), 18
incidence, 7
inhibitory allo-antibodies, 14, 15
laboratory findings, 5, 16
maintenance therapy, 19
management, 5, 14
pathology, 15
pdFVIII and rFVIII products, 15
physical examination, 3
recombinant coagulation factor VIIa (FVIIa), 19
Hemophilia B (HB)
activated prothrombin complex concentrate, 40
allergic and/or anaphylactic reactions, 43
bypassing agents, 40
cardiopulmonary stabilization, 36
case history, 25, 35
classification, 37
clinical presentation, 27
complications, 31, 32
concizumab, 32
desmopressin, 29
diagnosis, 29
differential diagnosis, 26, 36
epidemiology, 26
factor IX inhibitors, 42, 44–45
factor replacement, 30
family history, 38
Fitusiran (ALN-AT3SC), 32
FIX inhibitors, 41
FIX level, 32
fresh frozen plasma, 29
gene therapy, 32
genetic mutations, 38
genetic risk factors, 38
genetics, 27
Ig-E mediated mechanism, 38
inhibitor development, 37
laboratory evaluation, 36
low responding inhibitors, 42
Malmö protocol, 43
management, 26, 36
Missense mutations, 38
nephrotic syndrome, 43
Nijmegen modification, 36
non-genetic factors, 37
pathophysiology, 26, 37
prevention and treatment, 40
prophylaxis therapy, 30
rebalancing hemostasis, 32
recombinant coagulation factor VIIa (FVIIa), 40
therapeutic dosing and efficacy, 41
tissue factor pathway inhibitor (TFPI), 27
treatment strategies, 37, 40
Hermanksy-Pudlak syndrome (HPS), 208, 209
Heyde syndrome, 130

I

Immune thrombocytopenia (ITP)
case history, 141, 142, 151, 152
differential diagnosis, 142, 153
epidemiology, 144
first-line therapies, 154
HRQoL assessment tool, 157
laboratory findings, 145
management, 145–148
mucocutaneous bleeding symptoms, 143, 144

Immune thrombocytopenia (*cont.*)
   non-hematologic manifestation, 154
   oral immunosuppressive agents, 157
   pathophysiology, 144, 153
   physical examination, 143
   prevalence, 153
   primary immune thrombocytopenia, 143
   rituximab, 155
   second-line therapies, 155
   splenectomy, 156
   supportive care therapy, 152
   TPO-RA agents, 156
   treatment outcomes and follow-up, 157
Immune tolerance therapy (ITT), 18
Inherited bleeding disorders, 142
International Society on Thrombosis and Haemostasis (ISTH), 73
ISTH/SSC Joint Working Group's Bleeding Assessment Tool (ISTH-BAT), 88

M
Malmö protocol, 43
May-Hegglin anomaly, 197
MYH9-related disease (MYH-RD)
   antifibrinolytic medications, 200
   case history, 195
   clinical presentation, 197
   desmopressin, 200
   differential diagnosis, 196
   Dohle-like leukocyte inclusion bodies, 196
   laboratory findings, 197, 199
   local control, 199
   macrothrombocytopenia, 196
   May-Hegglin anomaly, 197
   platelet transfusions, 200
   preventative care, 199
   symptoms, 196
   treatment outcomes and follow-up, 201

P
Paris-Trousseau or Jacobsen syndrome, 213
Platelet granule disorders
   antifibrinolytic medications, 215
   case history, 205, 206
   clinical findings, 206
   desmopressin, 215
   diagnosis, 207
   differential diagnosis, 206
   epidemiology, 206
   local measures, 214
   platelet release disorder (*see* Platelet release disorder)
   platelet transfusions, 216
   preventative care, 214
   PSPD (*see* Platelet storage pool deficiency (PSPD))
   treatment outcomes and follow-up, 216
Platelet release disorder
   Paris-Trousseau or Jacobsen syndrome, 213
   platelet aggregation testing, 212
   Quebec platelet disorder (QPD), 214
Platelet storage pool deficiency (PSPD)
   α-PSPD, 210
   Arthrogryposis-Renal Dysfunction-Cholestasis (ARC) syndrome, 212
   Chediak-Higashi syndrome (CHS), 209
   δ-PSPD, 207, 208
   grey platelet syndrome (GPS), 210–212
   Hermanksy-Pudlak syndrome (HPS), 208, 209

idiopathic δ-PSPD, 209, 210
symptom, 207
X-linked thrombocytopenia, 212
Primary immune thrombocytopenia, 143

Q
Quebec platelet disorder (QPD), 214

S
Seven Treatment Evaluations Registry (STER), 63

T
Type 1 von Willebrand disease (VWD)
  adjunctive therapies
    antifibrinolytics, 95, 96
    desmopressin/DDAVP, 94, 95
  case history, 83
  clinical presentation, 85
  comprehensive care, 96
  differential diagnosis, 88–90
  history, 84
  laboratory findings, 89, 91, 93
  management, 84, 93
  pathophysiology, 85, 87
  replacement factors, 93
  type 1 C VWD, 87
  von Willebrand protein, 85–87
Type 2 von Willebrand disease (VWD)
  antifibrinolytic agents, 108
  bleeding management
    epistaxis, 110
    gastrointestinal (GI) tract, 110
    menorrhagia, 110
  bleeding symptoms, 100
  case history, 99
  clinical subtypes, 100
  D1472H variant, 106
  DDAVP, 108
  differential diagnosis, 102, 103
  functional sites and laboratory findings, 104
  genetic testing, 106
  GpIbM assay, 105
  initial laboratory evaluation, 103
  laboratory evaluation algorithm, 105
  laboratory findings, 103
  low-dose RIPA (LD-RIPA), 106
  management, 100
  multimer pattern analysis, 103, 104
  non-steroidal anti-inflammatory (NSAIDs), 107
  patient history, 101
  replacement therapy, 108
  ristocetin induced platelet aggregation (RIPA), 106
  therapeutic goal, 108
  treatment approaches, 109
  type 2A, 101
  type 2B, 101
  type 2M, 102
  type 2N, 102
  VWF, RCo assay, 104
Type 3 von Willebrand disease (VWD)
  alloantibodies, 122
  anti-coagulants, 122
  antifibrinolytics, 114
  case history, 113, 114
  clinical presentation, 115
  DDAVP based therapies, 114, 122
  differential diagnosis, 116
  dosing, 120–121
  epidemiology, 115
  factor VIII replacement, 114
  incidence, 115
  laboratory findings, 116, 117

Type 3 von Willebrand
 disease (VWD) (*cont.*)
 management and follow up,
 117–119
 non-steroidal anti-inflammatory
 (NSAIDs), 122
 prophylaxis, 123
 replacement therapy, 119
 treatment outcomes and
 follow-up, 123

V
von Willebrand disease (VWD), 27
von Willebrand factor (VWF), 6

W
Wiskott-Aldrich syndrome (WAS)
 case history, 161, 162
 curative options, 165
 differential diagnosis,
 163, 164
 epidemiology, 167
 gene therapy, 165
 hematopoietic stem cell
 transplantation
 (HSCT), 164
 inheritance/genetics, 167
 laboratory findings, 165, 166
 supportive management,
 164, 165
 treatment outcomes and
 follow-up, 168

X
X-linked thrombocytopenia, 212

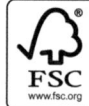

MIX
Papier aus verantwortungsvollen Quellen
Paper from responsible sources
FSC® C105338

If you have any concerns about our products,
you can contact us on
ProductSafety@springernature.com

In case Publisher is established outside the EU,
the EU authorized representative is:
**Springer Nature Customer Service Center GmbH
Europaplatz 3, 69115 Heidelberg, Germany**

Printed by Libri Plureos GmbH
in Hamburg, Germany